Surface
Anatom

Pocket tutor

Surface Anatomy

Richard Tunstall BMedSci (Hons) PhD FHEA
Associate Professor of Anatomy
University of Nottingham
Royal Derby Hospital

Nehal Shah MBBS BSc (Hons) MRCS FRCR
Specialist Registrar in Clinical Radiology
Leeds Teaching Hospitals Trust

pocket tutor

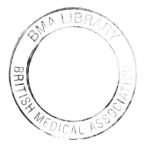

JP
medical
publishers

Published by JP Medical Ltd, 83 Victoria Street, London, SW1H 0HW, UK

Tel: +44 (0)20 3170 8910   Fax: +44 (0)20 3008 6180

Email: info@jpmedpub.com   Web: www.jpmedpub.com

ISBN: 978-1-907816-17-8

British Library Cataloguing in Publication Data
A catalogue record for this book is available from the British Library

Library of Congress Cataloging in Publication Data
A catalog record for this book is available from the Library of Congress

JP Medical Ltd is a subsidiary of Jaypee Brothers Medical Publishers (P) Ltd, New Delhi, India (www.jaypeebrothers.com).

Publisher:	Richard Furn
Development Editors:	Paul Mayhew, Alison Whitehouse
Design:	Designers Collective Ltd
Photography:	Sam Scott-Hunter

Indexed, typeset, printed and bound in India.

Foreword

The 'preclinical' years of my undergraduate course (i.e. years 1 and 2) in the mid 1960s were spent in lecture theatres, tutorial rooms and laboratories, and my timetable was filled exclusively with the basic medical sciences. Patients were encountered only very occasionally, in the artificial surroundings of a large lecture theatre. Anatomy was taught in enormous detail, often far beyond the level required of a medical student. Interestingly, surface anatomy was an afterthought, sometimes mentioned in a tutorial, rarely demonstrated on a student or model and hardly ever formally examined.

Modern medical curricula reflect the seismic shift that has occurred in thinking about medical education in the intervening years. Medical students now usually interact with patients from day 1, with basic medical science informing their clinical experiences to varying degrees throughout their course. In such a clinical context, it quickly becomes obvious that a working knowledge of topographical anatomy is essential for safe clinical practice. Using surface anatomy, i.e. knowing where anatomical structures lie under the skin by reference to prominent and consistent bony features, ligaments, tendons, muscle bellies or skin creases, students can learn to visualise and contextualise the topographical anatomy they need to know to examine their patients, interpret diagnostic images and perform basic interventional procedures such as catheter placement safely and effectively. They will also be able to appreciate the safe siting of surgical incisions when they observe in theatres or clinics – knowing where not to cut is every bit as important as knowing what may safely be incised.

For those who think that there is little new to learn in anatomy, it is worth noting that surface anatomy is currently under something of a spotlight. Recent evidence-based surface anatomy studies, in which surface features are related to measurements based on modern cross sectional images, rather than those based on cadaveric or early radiographic studies, indicate that we may have to reappraise some markings in the future to take account of variations according to age, body mass, posture, ethnicity or respiration. Richard Tunstall emphasises the need to bear variation in mind whenever surface positioning structures – a key point that reminds us that all patients are different.

This splendid pocket-sized book is packed with clinically relevant material designed to help medical students at all stages of their courses to learn and/or consolidate their knowledge of surface anatomy. Clinical insights add further relevance to the text. Readers should use the book to practise on themselves and on willing friends until they feel confident identifying bony landmarks and arterial pulses; palpating normal structures through intact skin; testing the range of movement of the joints. Sounds like an ideal way to improve communication skills as well as learn anatomy!

Susan Standring DSc FKC Hon FRCS
Emeritus Professor of Anatomy
King's College London
May 2012

Preface

A good knowledge of surface anatomy forms an essential part of safe and effective clinical practice for many healthcare specialities. When writing *Pocket Tutor Surface Anatomy* we took the broad view that surface anatomy includes clinically-relevant anatomy that can be located, related to, easily accessed or viewed via the surface of the body. With this in mind this book includes reference to movements, cutaneous innervation, referred pain, surgical/anaesthetic access and clinical conditions.

Throughout the book surface anatomy has been related to clinical practice, procedures and radiographs in order to provide context and aid understanding. Indeed, it is our view that surface anatomy is key to understanding and interpreting normal anatomy on medical images. Clear descriptions of location, appearance, reference landmarks and relationships are supported by a series of high quality overlaid images and tables. Chapter 1 introduces the principles of surface anatomy and overviews core anatomical terminology, palpation technique, movements and cutaneous innervation. Subsequent chapters (2-8) then review each main anatomical region in turn.

The book will be of benefit to students in anatomical, medical and healthcare disciplines and also to those in clinical practice, for example foundation doctors or surgical trainees. It can be used as a quick reference whilst in the clinic or teaching, but is equally adept at supporting more in-depth learning or revision. We have designed the book to either support current clinical anatomy courses and texts, or to be used as a stand-alone text.

The best way to learn surface anatomy is to get 'hands-on' with yourself, colleagues and patients. We hope this book serves as a useful and stimulating introduction.

Richard Tunstall
Nehal Shah
May 2012

How to learn surface anatomy

Surface anatomy is best learned via the examination and palpation of living subjects, the more the better. Remember also to cross-reference the information in this book with cadaveric specimens, sections and medical imaging. This will enhance your understanding of positions, variability and relationships. When surface positioning structures it is helpful to remember the following:

- Use prominent and consistent landmarks, such as bony features, ligaments, tendons and muscles, as reference points
- Observation, palpation, percussion and auscultation should be used to guide identification and placement
- Tissue manipulation, joint movement, muscle contraction and superficial vein occlusion can aid structure identification
- It is helpful and sometimes essential to mark/draw the locations of key structures and landmarks on a subject's skin
- Arteries, many of which are palpable, can act as a good guide to the surface location of neural structures
- Become familiar with the range of normal appearances since this makes the identification of abnormality easier

Contents

Acknowledgements

To my wife Liz, thank you for all of the encouragement, support, advice and good tea.

Thanks to Paul Mayhew and Richard Furn from JP Medical for their invaluable advice and guidance during this project, and to Richard Prime and Pete Wilder from Designers Collective Ltd for turning my anatomical sketches into artwork.

Introduction

The ability to locate anatomical structures via the surface of the body using observation, palpation and reference landmarks is an essential part of clinical medicine. A sound knowledge of surface anatomy enables a practitioner to understand the basis of physical examinations and medical procedures such as cannulation, biopsy, surgical incisions, local anaesthesia and intra-articular injection. Surface anatomy also assists with diagnostic reasoning and in the interpretation of medical images such as CT, MRI and ultrasound.

Measurements and variability

The descriptions within this book are based upon current observations, opinions and practice and the author's own observations. Although the surface positions of many structures are relatively consistent it should be noted that surface anatomy is subject to inter-individual variability and can change with body shape, size, condition and position.

   The measurements provided in this text should be used as a guide. A good practitioner needs to be aware of variability and should use observation, palpation, percussion, auscultation, nerve stimulation or ultrasound to further guide positing. In certain areas finger-breadth measurements are used since they often provide a useful quick measurement. These start with the tip of the index finger.

Ultrasound and surface anatomy

Ultrasound is increasingly being used by practitioners to help provide additional guidance during invasive procedures. It is also a useful tool when learning surface anatomy. It should be noted that ultrasound does not replace the need to learn surface anatomy, since a sound knowledge of surface anatomy and its potential variability is essential to the identification of structures on ultrasound.

Palpation Techniques

Efficient palpation technique forms an essential part of clinical practice. It is used to localise anatomical structures and landmarks, and to determine tissue structure and pathological change. As a general rule sides are compared, especially in suspected pathology. Tenderness should not normally be elicited upon palpation. Different techniques are used to palpate different tissue, regions and features (**Table 1.1**).

Tissue/feature	Palpation technique
Bone features and contour	Use the thumb or index finger in a stroking/circular action or to apply direct gentle pressure
Muscles tone, tenderness and texture	Use direct thumb pressure to assess tone then move it at 90° to the muscle fibres to assess texture and tenderness. Normally muscle tone allows the pressure of a palpating thumb before the tissue thickness is felt
Superficial tendons	Use a gentle pinch grip with the thumb and index finger. Working along the tendon aids identification
Deep tendons	Palpate at the bone attachment point using direct pressure from a thumb being worked in a small circle, then continue along the tendon working the thumb from side to side
Tendons sheaths	Place the tips of digits 2–4 along the tendon, without pressure, then ask the patient to repeatedly work the tendon. Crepitus feels like the crushing of a snowball
Ligaments	Palpate parallel to the ligaments fibres using light pressure via a thumb or index and middle finger
Joint lines	Press a finger or thumb into the space/groove between the two bones and trace it around the joint. The digit is worked over the joint line in an up-down action assessing for joint pathology and allowing for the palpation of muscles, tendons and ligaments crossing the joint
Vertebral column facet joints	With the patient prone the pisiform of one hand is placed onto the spinous process and, using the opposite hand, is pressed firmly anteriorly and immediately released so that the vertebra 'springs'. Tenderness is absent in unaffected joints. Cervical region joints can be moved by finger pressure alone.

Table 1.1 Palpation techniques.

1.1 The anatomical position and planes

The anatomical position

Within this book all positions, relationships and movements of body structures have been described in relation to the anatomical position. The anatomical position is the standard reference position of the body (**Figure 1.1**). When in the anatomical position the subject is standing upright with the:

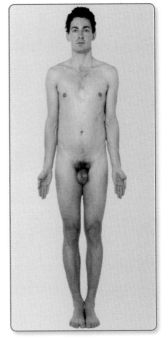

- Face, eyes, palms and toes facing forwards
- Upper limbs by the sides of the body
- Lower limbs, feet, fingers and toes together
- Thumbs resting against the lateral palms at 90° to the fingers

Relative positional terms

From the starting point of the anatomical position it is possible to describe the relative positions of structures using a standardised set of terms (**Figure 1.2** and **Table 1.2**).

Figure 1.1   The anatomical position.

Anatomical planes

From the anatomical position the body can be sectioned by three mutually perpendicular planes (**Figure 1.3** and **Table 1.3**).

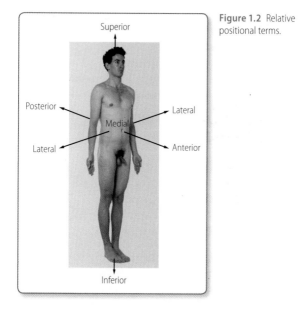

Figure 1.2 Relative positional terms.

Term	Relative position
Anterior	Toward the front of the body
Posterior	Toward the back of the body
Medial	Toward the midline
Lateral	To the left or right of the midline
Superior	Toward the top of the head
Inferior	Toward the soles of the feet
Cranial	Toward the head (cranium)
Caudal	Toward the tail (coccyx)
Distal	A point away from the origin of a structure/main body
Proximal	A point toward the origin of a structure/main body

Table 1.2 Relative positional terms.

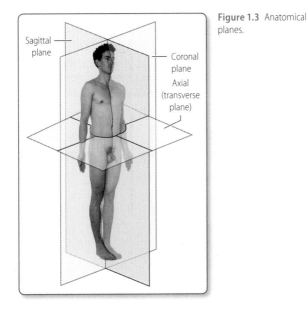

Figure 1.3 Anatomical planes.

Plane	Location
Sagittal	Passes vertically from anterior to posterior, separating the body into left and right sides
Coronal (frontal)	Passes vertically from left to right, separating the body into anterior and posterior parts
Axial (transverse)	Passes horizontally through the body separating it into superior and inferior parts
Oblique	Any plane that is neither sagittal, coronal nor axial

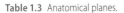

Table 1.3 Anatomical planes.

1.2 Anatomical movements

The movement of a joint or part of the body is described from the starting point of the anatomical position. A knowledge of joint movement is useful in surface anatomy since specified movements can aid structure identification and be required for clinical examination and procedures.

Flexion and extension

Flexion and extension occur in the sagittal plane (**Figures 1.4–1.14**).

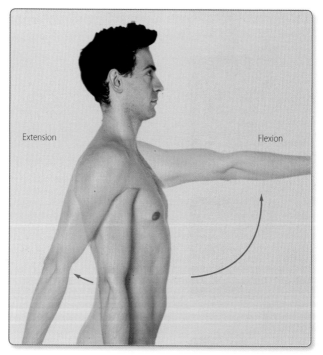

Figure 1.4 Shoulder extension and flexion.

- **Flexion** brings together two surfaces that were originally on the ventral surface of the embryo
- **Extension** moves apart two surfaces that were originally on the ventral surface of the embryo

Flexion moves most structures anteriorly whereas extension moves most structures posteriorly. The main exceptions to this occur at the knee, ankle, toes and thumb. For example, plantarflexion is the flexion movement of the feet or toes, dorsiflexion being the extension movement. Flexion of the thumb moves it across the palm in a coronal plane, and extension moves it in the opposite direction.

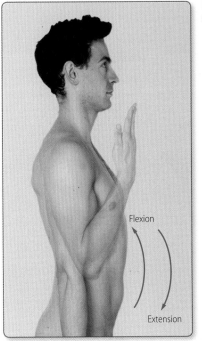

Figure 1.5 Elbow extension and flexion.

Flexion

Extension

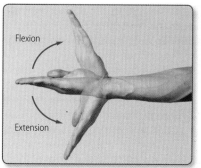

Figure 1.6 Wrist extension and flexion.

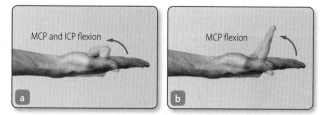

Figure 1.7 Digital flexion: (a) metacarpophalangeal and interphalangeal joints; (b) metacarpophalangeal joints.

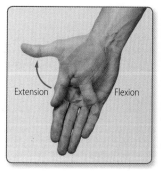

Figure 1.8 Thumb extension and flexion.

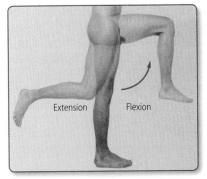

Figure 1.9 Hip extension and flexion.

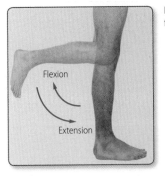

Figure 1.10 Knee extension and flexion.

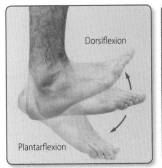

Figure 1.11 Ankle plantarflexion (flexion) and dorsiflexion (extension).

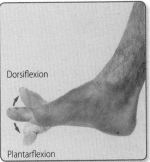

Figure 1.12 Toe dorsiflexion (extension) and plantarflexion (flexion).

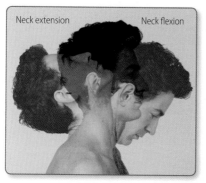

Figure 1.13 Neck extension and flexion.

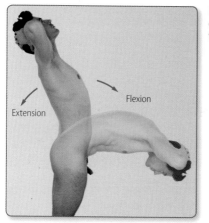

Figure 1.14 Vertebral column extension and flexion.

Abduction and adduction

Abduction and adduction occur in the coronal plane (**Figures 1.15–1.20**).

- **Abduction** moves a structure away from the median sagittal plane
- **Adduction** moves a structure closer to the median sagittal plane

The digits differ in that the movements take place in relation the 3rd digit in the hand and the 2nd digit in the foot. Abduction of the thumb moves it away from the palm in a sagittal plane, and adduction returns it to the anatomical position.

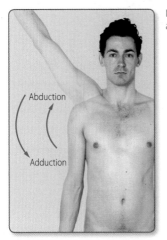

Figure 1.15 Shoulder abduction and adduction.

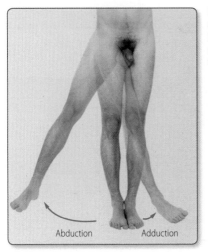

Figure 1.16 Hip abduction and adduction. Hip adduction can take place across the midline if opposite limb is avoided.

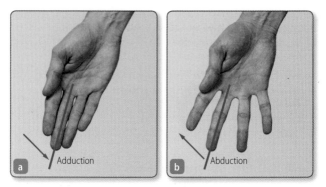

Figure 1.17 Finger abduction and adduction.

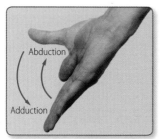

Figure 1.18 Thumb abduction and adduction.

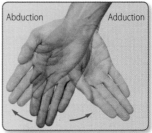

Figure 1.19 Wrist abduction and adduction.

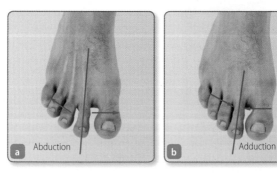

Figure 1.20 Toe (a) abduction and (b) adduction. The blue line represents the axis of abduction/adduction.

Rotation

Rotation occurs in the transverse plane (**Figures 1.21–1.24**).

- **Medial (internal) rotation** moves the anterior surface of a limb closer to the median sagittal plane
- **Lateral (external) rotation** moves the anterior surface of the limb away from the median sagittal plane
- **Axial rotation** of the vertebral column and atlanto-occipital joints enables turning of the head and body to the left or right

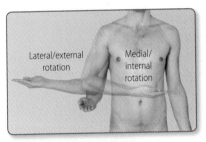

Figure 1.21 Shoulder rotation: lateral (external) and medial (internal) rotation.

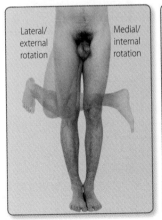

Figure 1.22 Hip rotation: medial (internal) and lateral (external) rotation.

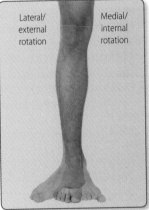

Figure 1.23 Knee rotation: lateral (external) and medial (internal) rotation.

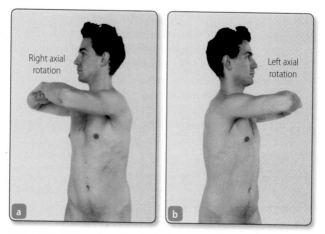

Figure 1.24 Axial rotation of the vertebral column.

Pronation and supination

In the forearm:

- **Pronation** rotates the radius medially around the ulna such that the palm of the hand faces posteriorly (**Figure 1.25**)
- **Supination** is the opposite movement: it returns the palm to the anatomical position

In the foot:

- **Pronation** lifts its lateral edge such that the sole face away from the median sagittal plane
- **Supination** lifts the medial edge such that the sole faces the median sagittal plane (**Figure 1.26**)

Foot pronation and supination is usually accompanied by foot abduction and adduction, respectively.

Inversion and eversion of the foot

- Inversion is a combination of adduction, supination and plantarflexion
- Eversion is a combination of abduction, pronation and dorsiflexion (**Figure 1.27**)

Both movements occur naturally when attempting to make the sole face medially or laterally with the foot lifted off the floor.

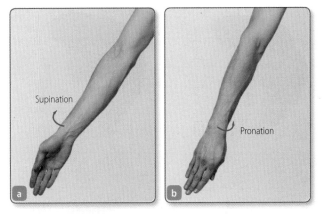

Figure 1.25 Forearm supination and pronation. (a) Supination brings to supine position. (b) Pronation brings forearm to prone position.

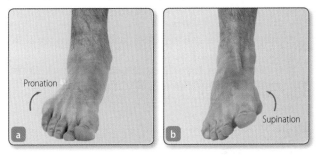

Figure 1.26 Foot pronation (a) and supination (b).

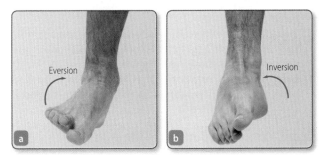

Figure 1.27 Foot eversion (a) and inversion (b).

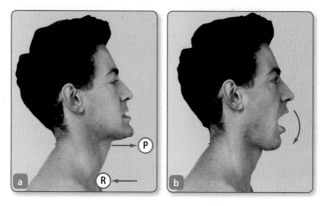

Figure 1.28 Mandibular movements: (a) protrusion (P) and retrusion (R).
(b) mandibular opening.

Mandibular movements
- **Protrusion** moves the mandible (and therefore the chin) anteriorly in a transverse plane
- **Retrusion** moves the mandible posteriorly back to the anatomical position (**Figure 1.28**)
  Mandibular opening combines protrusion and rotation.

Scapular movements
- **Protraction** moves the scapula anterolaterally around the thoracic wall, such as when reaching forward; **retraction** is the opposite posteromedial movement toward the vertebral column (**Figure 1.29**)
- **Elevation** moves the scapula superiorly on the thoracic wall, such as when shrugging the shoulder; **depression** is the opposite inferior movement (**Figure 1.30**)
- **External/lateral rotation** makes the glenoid fossa face superolaterally; **internal/medial rotation** is the opposite movement (**Figure 1.31**)

Opposition and reposition of the digits
Opposition is the pad-to-pad contact of the thumb and fingers; it involves a specialised movement of the thumb (**Figure 1.32**).

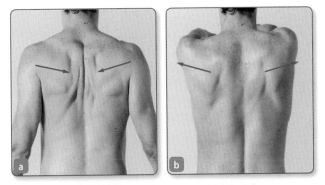

Figure 1.29 Scapular movements: (a) retraction and (b) protraction.

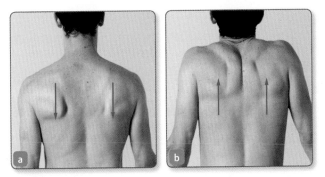

Figure 1.30 Scapular movements: (a) depression and (b) elevation.

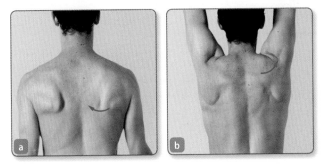

Figure 1.31 Scapular movements: (a) medial (internal) rotation and (b) lateral (external) rotation.

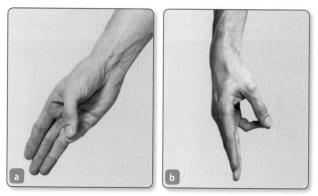

Figure 1.32 Thumb opposition: (a) anterior view and (b) lateral view.

It is essential for fine dexterous activities such as writing and buttoning clothes. **Reposition** returns the thumb to the anatomical position.

Lateral flexion

Lateral flexion is a lateral movement of the vertebral column in a coronal plane, which results in the head moving away from the midline (**Figures 1.33** and **1.34**).

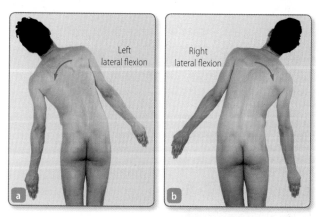

Figure 1.33 Lateral flexion of the vertebral column: (a) left and (b) right.

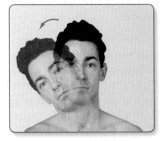

Figure 1.34 Lateral flexion of the neck.

Eye movements

The eyes move around three different axes. The movements of abduction–adduction, elevation–depression, and combinations of these are easily observed (**Figure 1.35**). Most eye movements are conjugate, except for convergence, in which both eyes adduct to enable observation of nearby objects (**Figure 1.36**).

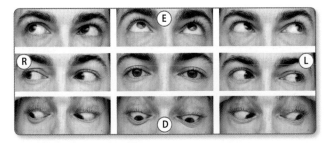

Figure 1.35 Eye movements. Ⓔ Elevation, Ⓓ depression, Ⓛ left-eye abduction and right-eye adduction, Ⓡ right-eye abduction and left-eye adduction.

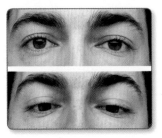

Figure 1.36 Eye movement: convergence.

1.3 Sensory innervation

A knowledge of cutaneous innervation patterns is important when mapping out sensory losses because it provides clues as to the location of damage. Cutaneous innervation can be defined by dermatome (**Figures 1.37** and **1.38**), which equates to the area of skin innervated by a single spinal nerve, or by cutaneous nerve area (**Figures 1.39** and **1.40**), which equates to the area of skin innervated by a named peripheral nerve. Cutaneous nerves can innervate skin across one or more dermatomes. As a general rule:

- Dermatomal sensory losses occur following damage to spinal nerves or their ventral rami
- Cutaneous nerve area sensory losses tend to occur as a result of distal nerve lesions caused by surgical incisions or laceration
- Many cutaneous nerves run close to superficial limb veins and are therefore at risk of injury during cannulation and vein removal

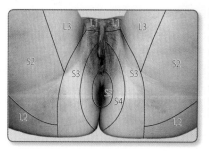

Figure 1.37 An evidence-based pelvic dermatome map. Based on Lee MWL, McPhee RW, Stringer MD. An Evidence-Based Approach to Human Dermatomes. Clinical Anatomy 2008;21:363–373.

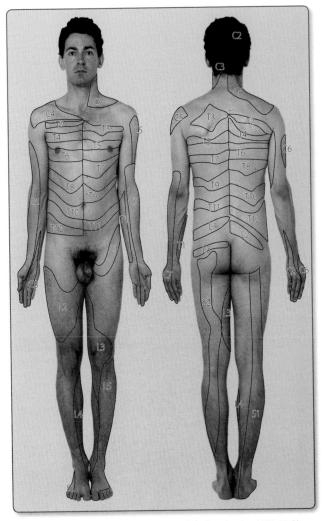

Figure 1.38 An evidence-based dermatome map. Based on Lee MWL, McPhee RW, Stringer MD. An evidence-based approach to human dermatomes. Clinical Anatomy 2008;21:363–373.

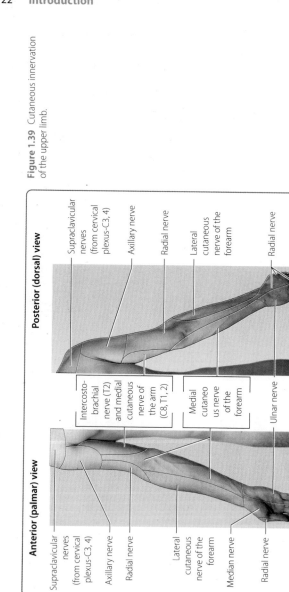

Figure 1.39 Cutaneous innervation of the upper limb.

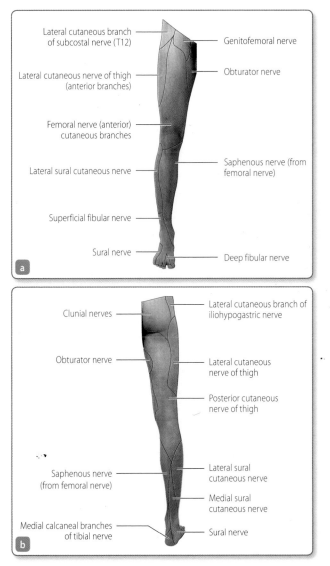

Figure 1.40 Cutaneous innervation of the lower limb: (a) anterior view and (b) posterior view.

Thorax

The thorax is the superior part of the trunk, located between the neck and abdomen. The region is surrounded by the thoracic wall, which is formed by the ribs, costal cartilages, intercostal muscles, skin, fascia and 12 thoracic vertebrae. The thoracic wall encloses the thoracic cavity, which extends from the thoracic inlet superiorly to the diaphragm inferiorly. The thorax contains the heart, lungs, associated vasculature and nerves, oesophagus, thymus and tracheobronchial tree. The mediastinum is the central region of the thorax located between the lungs, diaphragm, vertebral column and thoracic inlet.

Variability

The surface markings stated in this chapter are representative of an average-sized supine patient during quiet breathing. Remember that percussion, palpation, auscultation and ultrasound guidance can be used to further guide surface placement of underlying structures. The surface markings of thoracic viscera may vary depending on:

- Body position and associated gravity-induced changes
- Disease states, e.g. chronic obstructive pulmonary disease
- Deep inspiration/expiration
- Body mass

Function

The thoracic wall serves as an attachment point for muscles of the upper limb, back and abdominal wall, protects the thoracic viscera and assists in the mechanism of breathing and venous return to the heart. The inferior region of the thoracic wall together with the diaphragm and costodiaphragmatic recess cover and protect several organs of the abdominal cavity, which will be considered in Chapter 3.

2.1 Bony landmarks, joints and cartilages

Thoracic inlet

The thoracic inlet is an anteroinferiorly angled imaginary plane that is bordered by rib 1, vertebrae T1 and the sternal notch (**Figure 2.1**). The inlet opens into the superior thorax and mediastinum. The spinous process of C7 (vertebrae prominens) is the most prominent in the lower neck and overlies the vertebral body of T1.

Sternum

The sternum sits anteriorly in the midline where it is palpable (**Figure 2.1**). It is formed, from superior to inferior, by the

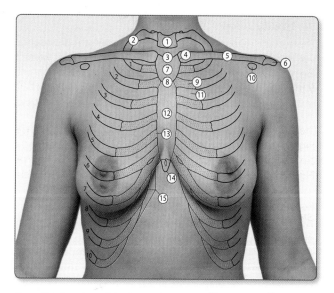

Figure 2.1 Osteology of the anterior thoracic wall. ① T1 vertebra, ② 1st rib, ③ sternal notch of manubrium, ④ sternoclavicular joint, ⑤ clavicle, ⑥ acromion, ⑦ manubrium, ⑧ sternal angle (manubriosternal joint), ⑨ 2nd costal cartilage, ⑩ coracoid process, ⑪ 2nd intercostal space, ⑫ sternal body, ⑬ sternocostal joint, ⑭ xiphoid process, ⑮ costal margin.

manubrium, body and xiphoid process. The sternal/jugular notch of the manubrium is palpable on its superior surface between the clavicles. Posterior palpation at the notch should reveal the trachea in the midline. The sternal body is a long plate of bone located inferior to the manubrium. The xiphoid process is located inferiorly and can protrude into the abdominal wall muscles. The 7th costal cartilage lies lateral to the xiphoid process. Sternal features can be used to identify vertebral levels (**Table 2.1**).

Clavicle and coracoid process

The clavicle is palpable and visible on the upper thorax between the acromion and manubrium (**Figure 2.1**). Its medial end forms the lateral border of the sternal notch and joins the manubrium at the prominent sternocla-vicular joint. The coracoid process is an anteriorly point-ing bony prominence of the scapula that forms a palpable rounded mass ~ 2 cm inferior to the lateral clavicle.

Clinical insight

Although the sternoclavicular joint is easily palpable and accessible, CT guidance is often used during aspiration and injection to prevent entry into the superior mediastinum and damage to pleura or great vessels.

Ribs

The ribs articulate with the thoracic vertebrae posteriorly (**Figure 2.2**) and curve anteroinferiorly around the thorax to join their respective costal cartilage on the anterior thoracic wall (**Figure 2.1**). Knowledge of a rib angulation aids radiographic

Sternal feature	Vertebral level
Sternal notch	T2
Manubrium	T2–T4
Sternal angle	T4/T5
Sternal body	T5–T8
Xiphoid process	T9

Table 2.1 Vertebral levels marked by the sternal features.

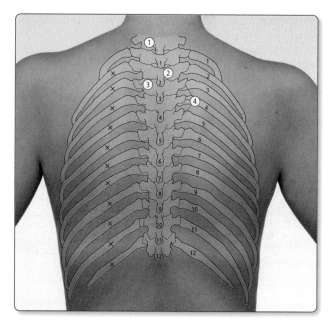

Figure 2.2 Osteology of the posterior thoracic wall. ① C7 spinous process, ② T1 spinous process, ③ T3 transverse process, ④ costotransverse joints, **x** rib angle. The thoracic vertebrae and ribs are numbered 1–12.

identification, for example, the posterior part of a rib appears to curve inferolaterally and is the most visible part (**Figure 2.3**). The angle of the rib is palpated posteriorly, a few centimetres lateral to the vertebral spinous processes. The angle is a useful marker for the lateral cutaneous nerves and vessels, which emerge just lateral to it and can be anaesthetised in the region.

Being able to count ribs is important for landmarking and safe thoracic access. Ribs 4–10 can be palpated in the midaxillary line starting with rib 4 at the skin of the axillary floor. Rib 10 is continuous with the costal margin. The free lateral ends of ribs 11 and 12, the floating/free ribs, can be palpated

Clinical insight

A thoracotomy incision at the 5th rib level enables upper thoracic access, whereas at the 7th rib level it enables oesophageal and diaphragmatic access.

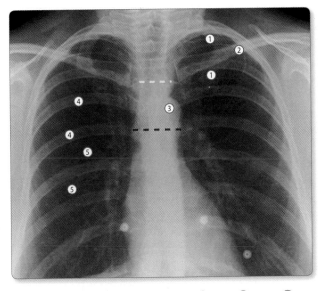

Figure 2.3 Postero-anterior thoracic radiograph. (1) 1st rib, (2) clavicle, (3) aortic arch, (4) posterior part of rib, (5) anterior part of rib, sternal plane (red dashed line), sternal notch (yellow dashed line).

posteriorly in lean individuals and can be traced medially to help identify the T11 and T12 vertebrae.

Costal cartilages and costal margin

The costal cartilages

These connect the distal parts of ribs 1–10 to the sternum or adjacent costal cartilage (**Figure 2.2**). In lean individuals the cartilage of ribs 1–7 vertebrosternal can be identified at the sternum and serve as useful markers of underlying structures. The cartilages pass medially, or superomedially, to the sternum and can be identified on radiographs by their direction of travel and relative radiolucency.

Costal margin This refers to the free inferior border of the anterior and lateral thoracic cage formed by the distal ends of costal cartilages 7–10. It can be palpated inferolaterally from the xiphisternum to rib 10, and is a useful landmark in abdominal examination.

Intercostal spaces

The intercostal spaces are located between adjacent ribs/costal cartilages, and are numbered according to the superiorly located rib (**Figure 2.2**). The second costal cartilage, located lateral to the sternal angle, acts as a useful landmark when counting intercostal spaces. The first intercostal space sits superiorly and the second sits inferiorly.

2.2 Muscles

Muscles of the thorax act on the ribs, upper limb or both (**Figure 2.4**).

Pectoralis major This is attached to the medial half of clavicle, costal cartilages 1–6 and the corresponding sternum, and passes laterally to attach to the upper humerus. It is seen and palpated on the anterior thoracic wall, and its free inferior border forms the anterior axillary fold along which the tail of the breast is palpated.

Pectoralis minor This is located deep to pectoralis major. It passes from ribs 3–5 in the midclavicular line to the coracoid process of the scapula, which is palpable beneath the lateral clavicle.

Subclavius This is located between the first rib and the inferior surface the clavicle, to around its middle third. It separates the subclavian vessels from the clavicle, and can protect them in a clavicular fracture. Subclavius is at risk of damage during catheter insertion into the subclavian vein via an infraclavicular route.

Intercostal muscles These are located between the ribs/cartilages of each intercostal space and are palpated as a soft depression. There are three layers of intercostal muscles ordered external, internal and innermost intercostal, from superficial to deep. The muscles can be incised to access the thorax.

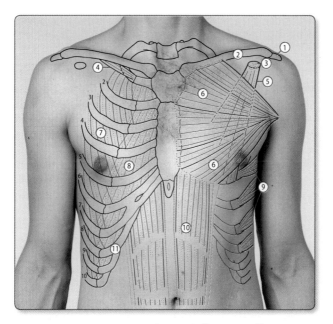

Figure 2.4 Muscles of the anterior thoracic wall. ① Acromion, ② clavicle, ③ coracoid process, ④ subclavius, ⑤ pectoralis minor, ⑥ pectoralis major, ⑦ external intercostal muscle, ⑧ internal intercostal muscle deep to external intercostal membrane, ⑨ serratus anterior, ⑩ rectus abdominis, ⑪ costal margin.

Serratus anterior This arises as fleshy strips from the upper eight ribs around the midaxillary line. The lower five strips can normally be palpated. It passes under the scapula and attaches to its medial border. Injury to the long thoracic nerve paralyses the muscle resulting in scapula winging.

Rectus abdominis This is a paired midline strap muscle, passing from the pubic symphysis and crest to the xiphoid process and costal cartilages 5–7. In lean patients its segmented appearance is visible. Its function and strength can be examined by getting the supine patient to raise their head/flex their neck.

The diaphragm This attaches to the lower border of the thoracic cage and arches superiorly into the thorax. During quiet respiration it reaches the level of the xiphisternal joint/5th rib in the midclavicular line.

2.3 Lines and folds

Vertical lines

Several vertical lines can be drawn across the thoracic wall (**Figures 2.5** and **2.6**). These lines can serve as marker points for underlying structures and can help demarcate safe zones for invasive procedures.

- The midclavicular line passes vertically through the midpoint of the clavicle. It serves as a marker point for both thoracic and abdominal viscera and is used to divide the abdomen into regions
- The midsternal line and midvertebral lines pass vertically along the midline of the anterior and posterior surfaces of the body, respectively
- The paravertebral line passes vertically down the sides of the vertebral bodies

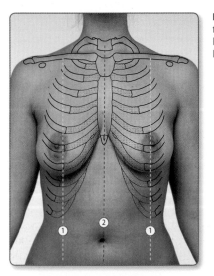

Figure 2.5 Anterior thoracic wall: vertical body lines. ① midclavicular line, ② midsternal line.

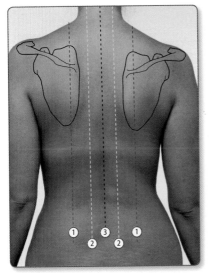

Figure 2.6 Posterior thoracic wall: vertical body lines. ① scapular line, ② paravertebral line, ③ midvertebral line.

- The scapular lines pass vertically through the inferior angle of the scapula

Axillary lines and folds

Axillary lines and folds (**Figure 2.7**) help position nerves, lymph nodes, breast tissue and planes for instrument/trocar insertion. The axillary folds are best seen and palpated with the upper limb in resisted adduction such as when pressing the hands onto the hips during breast examination. Thoracentesis is performed around the midaxillary line within a 'safe triangle/ zone' located between the anterior and posterior axillary folds and superior to a horizontal line drawn just above the nipple (**Figure 2.8**).

Midaxillary line

The midaxillary line passes vertically down the lateral thoracic wall from the apex of the axilla. The inferior limit of the lung sits on the line at the 8th rib and the costodiaphragmatic recess

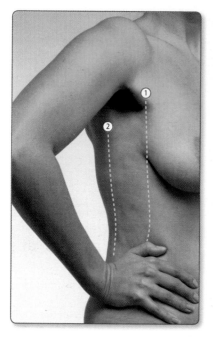

Figure 2.7 Lateral thoracic wall: axillary lines and folds. ① Anterior axillary fold and line, ② Posterior axillary fold and line.

extends between the 8th and 10th ribs on the line and overlies abdominal viscera.

Anterior axillary line and fold

The anterior axillary line passes vertically inferiorly from the anterior axillary fold. The anterior axillary fold is the free inferior border of the anterior axillary wall, which is formed by the tail of the breast overlying the inferolateral border of pectoralis major as it spans from the thorax to the humerus. The tail of the breast and lymph nodes must be examined in this region.

Posterior axillary line and fold

The posterior axillary line passes vertically inferiorly from the posterior axillary fold. The posterior axillary fold is the free

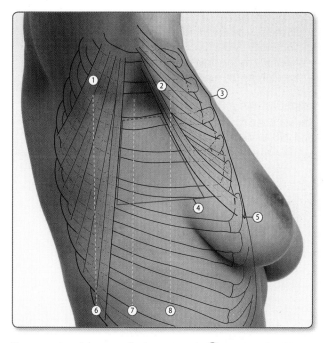

Figure 2.8 Lateral thoracic wall: safe zone/triangle. ① Posterior axillary fold, ② anterior axillary fold, ③ sternal angle, ④ borders of the safe triangle/zone for thoracentesis (red outline), ⑤ xiphoid process, ⑥ posterior axillary line, ⑦ midaxillary line, ⑧ anterior axillary line.

inferior border of the posterior axillary wall, which is formed by the inferior borders of latissimus dorsi and teres minor as they span from the thorax and scapula to the humerus.

2.4 Mediastinum

Location and borders

The mediastinum is the central region of the thoracic cavity located between the lungs. It mainly contains cardiovascular structures, which can be examined via the surface and identified on radiographs. The mediastinum is bordered (**Figure 2.9**):

- Anteriorly by the sternum
- Posteriorly by the thoracic vertebrae
- Superiorly by the thoracic inlet
- Inferiorly by the diaphragm
- Laterally by the lungs

Superior and inferior mediastinum

The sternal plane (T4/T5) divides the mediastinum into superior and inferior parts (**Figures 2.3** and **2.9**):

- The **superior mediastinum** is located between the thoracic inlet superiorly, the sternal plane inferiorly, the manubrium

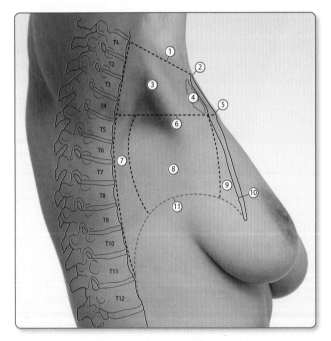

Figure 2.9 Lateral view of mediastinum. (1) Plane of thoracic inlet, (2) sternal notch, (3) superior mediastinum, (4) thymus gland, (5) sternal angle (manubriosternal joint), (6) sternal plane, (7) posterior mediastinum, (8) middle mediastinum, (9) anterior mediastinum, (10) xiphisternal joint, (11) diaphragm.

anteriorly and the T1–T4 vertebrae posteriorly. It contains the great vessels, arch of the aorta, superior vena cava and thymus

- The **inferior mediastinum** is located between the sternal plane superiorly, the sternal body anteriorly, the diaphragm inferiorly (marked by the xiphisternal junction) and the T5–T12 vertebrae posteriorly

Anterior, middle and posterior mediastinum

The inferior mediastinum can be subdivided into the anterior, middle and posterior mediastinum (**Figure 2.9**):

- The **anterior mediastinum** is located between the sternum and the fibrous pericardium. It contains the internal thoracic vessels and sometimes the thymus gland
- The **middle mediastinum** is mostly surrounded by the fibrous pericardium. It contains the heart and pericardial cavity and also includes the ascending aorta and lower part of the superior vena cava
- The **posterior mediastinum** is located between the fibrous pericardium, lower thoracic vertebrae and diaphragm. It contains the oesophagus, descending aorta and thoracic duct

Fluid/blood accumulation in the pericardial cavity can cause cardiac tamponade. Pericardiocentesis is performed to aspirate the fluid. A needle is inserted just inferior to the xiphoid/costal margin and directed towards the left shoulder thus penetrating the diaphragm and entering the pericardial cavity in the middle mediastinum.

2.5 Neurovasculature and lymphatics

Dermatomes

The thoracic dermatomes curve around the thoracic wall from the midvertebral to the midsternal line (**Figure 1.38**). Each dermatome is innervated by the spinal nerve travelling in the underlying intercostal space, although adjacent dermatomes overlap considerably. Three landmark dermatomes can be identified on the anterior thorax:

- C4 immediately below the clavicle

- T2 at the sternal angle
- T6 at the xiphisternum

Intercostal neurovascular bundles

The main intercostal neurovascular bundles are located below the superior rib of each intercostal space and between the internal and innermost intercostal muscles (**Figure 2.10**). The bundle is arranged vein, artery and nerve, from superior to inferior, and is vulnerable to damage during invasive procedures resulting in sensory loss, intercostal muscle paralysis and/or haemothorax. An accessory intercostal bundle can branch from the main bundle between the angle of the rib and posterior axillary line, then cross the space and run along the lower rib. Incising the intercostal space just above the superior border of a rib helps minimise the risk of damage to either bundle.

Cutaneous nerves and arteries

- **Lateral cutaneous branches** of intercostal nerves together with the lateral cutaneous arteries arise between the angle of the rib and the midaxillary line, with many emerging close to the latter

- **Anterior cutaneous branches** of intercostal nerves together with the anterior perforating arteries penetrate the intercostal muscles and pectoralis major ~ 1 cm lateral to the sternum to supply the overlying tissues

Long thoracic nerve

The long thoracic nerve passes inferiorly between the midaxillary and posterior axillary lines to the level of rib 8. The nerve

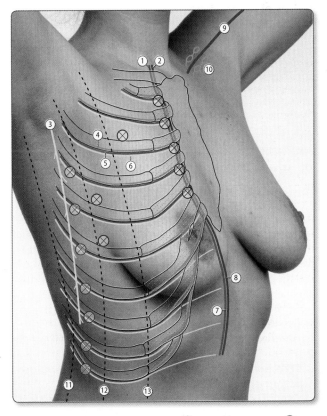

Figure 2.10 Thoracic wall neurovasculature. ① Internal thoracic artery, ② internal thoracic vein, ③ long thoracic nerve, ④ intercostal vein, ⑤ intercostal artery, ⑥ intercostal nerve, ⑦ superior epigastric artery, ⑧ superior epigastric vein, ⑨ cephalic vein, ⑩ deltopectoral lymph nodes, ⑪ posterior axillary line, ⑫ midaxillary line, ⑬ anterior axillary line, Ⓧ point of lateral cutaneous nerve and artery branch emergence, Ⓧ point of anterior cutaneous nerve and artery branch emergence, purple Ⓧ point of incision/entry for thoracentesis.

sits superficial to serratus anterior where it is vulnerable to damage in axillary surgery or during insertion of chest drains or trochars. Damage results in scapula winging.

Clinical insight

Midline division of the sternum from the jugular notch to xiphisternum (median sternotomy) permits access to the heart and avoids damage to internal thoracic vessels and anterior cutaneous neurovasculature.

Internal thoracic artery and vein

The internal thoracic artery and vein are located on the inner surface of the anterior thoracic wall, ~ 1 cm lateral to the edges of the sternum. Both vessels continue inferiorly into the rectus sheath as the superior epigastric vessels and can be harvested for coronary artery bypass grafting and viewed on arteriograms.

Lymphatics

Axillary lymph nodes These are located within the axilla and receive lymph from the upper limb, the majority of breast and the trunk wall above the umbilicus (**Figure 2.11**). Lymph drains toward central, apical then supraclavicular nodes. Nodes can enlarge due to infection or cancer. Axillary nodes are grouped and palpated according to position:

- **Lateral (humeral) nodes** sit anterolaterally close to the axillary vein and humerus
- **Anterior (pectoral) nodes** sit along the inner surface of the anterior axillary fold
- **Posterior (subscapular) nodes** sit along the inner surface of the posterior axillary fold
- **Central nodes** sit centrally within the axillary fat
- **Apical nodes** sit high in the axillary apex, close to ribs 1 and 2

Parasternal lymph nodes These are located on the inner surface of anterior thoracic wall alongside the internal thoracic artery. The nodes drain the breast tissue, and the thoracic and abdominal walls.

Deltopectoral lymph nodes These are located alongside the cephalic vein in the deltopectoral groove, just inferior to the clavicle. They receive lymph from the radial side of the limb and parts of the anterolateral thoracic wall and breast.

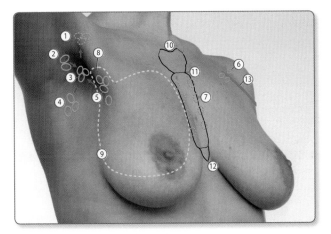

Figure 2.11 Axillary and thoracic wall lymph nodes. ① Apical nodes, ② lateral (humeral) nodes, ③ central nodes, ④ posterior (subscapular) nodes, ⑤ anterior (pectoral) nodes, ⑥ deltopectoral nodes, ⑦ parasternal nodes, ⑧ anterior axillary fold and axillary tail of breast, ⑨ border of base of the breast, ⑩ sternal notch, ⑪ sternal angle/plane, ⑫ xiphoid process, ⑬ cephalic vein.

Cephalic vein

The cephalic vein of the upper limb passes along the deltopectoral groove between deltoid and pectoralis major (**Figures 2.10** and **2.11**). The upper end of the deltopectoral groove represents a point for catheter insertion into the subclavian vein and contains deltopectoral lymph nodes, which can enlarge in upper limb/breast infection or breast cancer.

2.6 Viscera

Breast

Size, shape and position

The size, shape and position of female breast tissue is variable. The base/bed of the breast, however, sits anterior to pectoralis major and serratus anterior in a consistent position extending from rib 2 superiorly to rib 6 inferiorly and from the lateral sternal border medially to the midaxillary line laterally (**Figure 2.12**). The axillary tail (of Spence) of breast extends

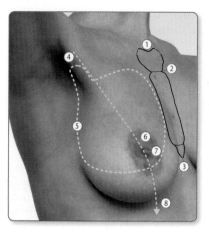

Figure 2.12 Female breast. (1) Sternal notch, (2) sternal angle, (3) xiphoid process, (4) axillary tail of breast, (5) border of base of the breast, (6) areola, (7) nipple, (8) mammary ridge (milk line).

superolaterally into the axilla and during breast examination is palpated along the inferolateral border of pectoralis major.

Areola and nipple

The areola is the darkened raised area of skin surrounding the nipple (**Figure 2.12**). It is covered in sweat and sebaceous areolar (Montgomery) glands, which can become infected and inflamed.

The male nipple sits over the 4th intercostal space, close to the midclavicular line, whereas female nipple position varies with age and breast size. The female nipple receives ~ 15–20 lactiferous ducts the openings of which can be seen when infected or lactating.

Clinical insight

The breast should not move during pectoral muscle contraction, elicited by pressing the hands into the hips. Movement suggests an underlying pathology resulting in breast adherence to underlying tissue.

Clinical insight

Supernumerary nipples can be present anywhere along the mammary ridge/ milk line, which runs from the anterior axillary fold through the nipple to the pubic tubercle.

Lungs and pleura

Pleura and costodiaphragmatic recess

Knowledge of the position of the pleural borders guides

physical examinations and helps prevent damage/pneumothorax associated with invasive procedures. Two layers of pleural membrane surround the lungs. Visceral pleura covers the lung surface and parietal pleura lines the inner thoracic wall, the superior diaphragm and the outer surface of the mediastinum. The costodiaphragmatic recess is located between the lower thoracic wall and the periphery of the diaphragm (**Figure 2.13**). It occupies the two rib/costal cartilage difference between the lower limits of the parietal pleura and the visceral pleura-covered lung and is therefore parietal-pleura lined.

Lung and pleural borders

The borders of the lung and pleura can be mapped out on the thoracic wall (**Figures 2.13** and **2.14**). The lung apex and its pleural coverings are located ~ 2–3 cm above the

> ### Clinical insight
>
> The costodiaphragmatic recess overlies the liver and kidney. It can therefore be penetrated during biopsy and surgical access, which may cause pneumothorax.

middle of the medial third of the clavicle where they are at risk during central venous cannulation. The lung and its pleural coverings then pass to the midsternal line at the sternal angle level. On the right both continue inferiorly to the 6th costal cartilage level whereas on the left both the lung and pleura move laterally by ~ 4 cm at the 4th costal cartilage to accommodate the heart, and then then pass inferiorly to the 6th costal cartilage.

At the lower sternal level the surface markings of both lungs and their parietal pleura then separate as they curve postero-laterally around the thoracic wall as shown in **Table 2.2**.

	Pleural location	Lung location
Midclavicular line	8th costal cartilage	6th rib
Midaxillary line	10th rib	8th rib
Scapular line	12th rib	10th rib
Paravertebral line	T12 spinous process	T10 spinous process

Table 2.2 Surface markings of the lung and parietal pleura. The costodiaphragmatic recess occupies the gap between them.

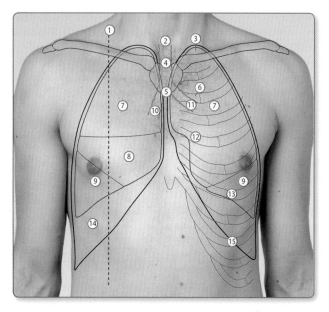

Figure 2.13 Anterior surface markings of the lungs and pleura. ① Midclavicular line, ② trachea, ③ lung apex, ④ sternal notch, ⑤ sternal angle/plane and tracheal bifurcation, ⑥ 2nd costal cartilage, ⑦ superior lobe of lung, ⑧ middle lobe of lung, ⑨ inferior lobe of lung, ⑩ right main bronchus, ⑪ left main bronchus, ⑫ 4th costal cartilage, ⑬ 6th rib in the midclavicular line, ⑭ costodiaphragmatic recess, ⑮ 8th costal cartilage in the midclavicular line.

Both the parietal pleura and lung then pass superiorly together along the paravertebral line to meet the surface markings at the apex. The pleura is vulnerable to damage at the lung apex and posteriorly at T12.

Lung lobes and fissures

The lungs are divided into lobes by fissures. The right lung has three lobes (superior, middle and inferior) and the left two lobes (superior and inferior) (**Figures 2.13** and **2.14**). Respiratory system examination requires different areas of each lobe to be examined. The right middle lobe is best heard in the

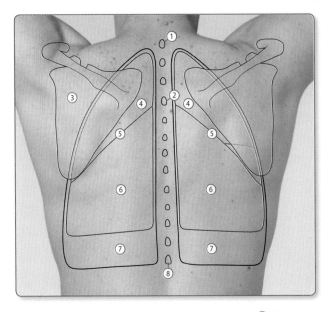

Figure 2.14 Posterior surface markings of the lungs and pleura. ① C7 Spinous process, ② T3 Spinous process, ③ Scapula, ④ Superior lobe of lung, ⑤ Oblique fissure following medial border of scapula of abducted limb, ⑥ Inferior lobe of lung, ⑦ Costodiaphragmatic recess , ⑧ T12 spinous process.

axillary region and bronchial breath sounds can normally be heard centrally over the main bronchi but not over the lung.

Oblique fissure Both lungs have an oblique fissure that curves around the thoracic wall from the spinous process of T3 posteriorly (overlies T4 vertebral level) to the 6th costal cartilage anteriorly between the midclavicular line and sternum. The medial border of the scapula of an abducted upper limb provides a good approximation of the oblique fissure.

Horizontal fissure The right lung has a horizontal fissure that passes from the 4th costal cartilage at the sternum to the 4th rib in the midaxillary line. It meets the oblique fissure near to the posterior axillary line (**Figure 2.15**).

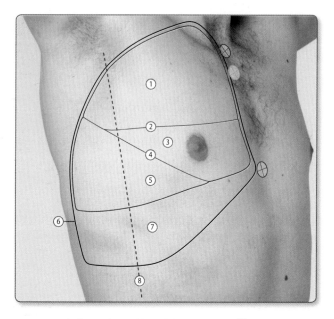

Figure 2.15 Surface markings of the right lung and pleura. ① Superior lobe of lung, ② horizontal fissure, ③ middle lobe of lung, ④ oblique fissure, ⑤ inferior lobe of lung, ⑥ parietal pleura, ⑦ costodiaphragmatic recess overlying liver, ⑧ midaxillary line, ⓧ sternal notch, ⓧ sternal angle, ⓧ xiphoid process.

Tracheobronchial tree

The trachea originates at vertebral level C6 inferior to the cricoid cartilage and passes inferiorly to bifurcate into the right and left main bronchi at the level of the sternal angle (vertebral level T4–T5). It is palpable in the midline above the sternal notch. The right main bronchus follows a relatively vertical course to the lung hilum at vertebral level T5–T7 (costal cartilages 3–5), whereas the left main bronchus follows a more horizontal route to the hilum. Knowledge of the position of tracheobronchial tree structures aids their examination and identification on medical images (**Figures 2.16** and **2.17**).

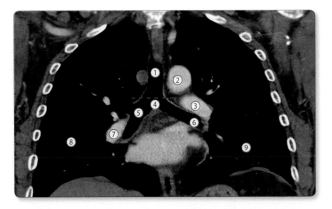

Figure 2.16 Coronal thoracic CT. ① Trachea, ② aortic arch, ③ left pulmonary artery, ④ carina, ⑤ right main bronchus, ⑥ left main bronchus, ⑦ right pulmonary artery, ⑧ right lung, ⑨ left lung, sternal plane (red dashed line).

Heart

Heart borders The heart occupies the middle mediastinum (**Figures 2.17** and **2.18**). Its projection onto the anterior thoracic wall can be mapped out between four points (**Table 2.3**).

Clinical insight

Tracheal deviation from the midline can indicate a pathology pushing it (tension pneumothorax/effusion/tumour) or pulling it (lung fibrosis/collapse) to one side.

Point	Surface position	Chamber/feature
Upper right	Right 3rd costal cartilage ~1 cm lateral to sternum	Right atrium and superior vena cava
Lower right	Right 6th costal cartilage ~1 cm lateral to sternum	Right atrium and inferior vena cava
Upper left	Left 2nd costal cartilage ~1 cm lateral to the sternum	Auricle of left atrium and pulmonary trunk
Lower left/ apex	Left 5th intercostal space just medial to the midclavicular line	Apex and left ventricle

Table 2.3 Surface markings of the heart on the anterior thoracic wall.

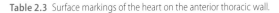

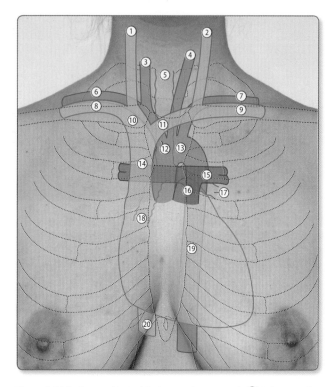

Figure 2.17 Surface markings of the heart and great vessels. ① Right internal jugular vein, ② left internal jugular vein, ③ right common carotid artery, ④ left common carotid artery, ⑤ trachea, ⑥ right subclavian artery, ⑦ left subclavian artery, ⑧ right subclavian vein, ⑨ left subclavian vein, ⑩ right brachiocephalic vein, ⑪ left brachiocephalic vein, ⑫ brachiocephalic trunk, ⑬ arch of aorta, ⑭ superior vena cava, ⑮ left pulmonary artery, ⑯ pulmonary trunk, ⑰ left main bronchus, ⑱ right main bronchus, ⑲ descending aorta, ⑳ inferior vena cava.

Using these points, the right heart border extends between the right upper and lower points and is formed by the right atrium, the left border extends between the left upper and lower points and is mostly formed by the left ventricle. The inferior heart border joins the lower left and lower right points

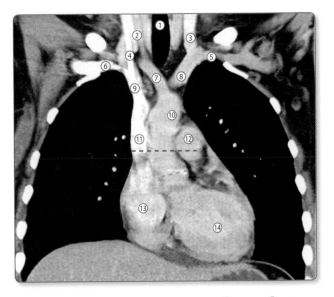

Figure 2.18 Coronal CT of the heart and great vessels. ①Trachea, ② right common carotid artery, ③ left internal jugular vein, ④ right internal jugular vein, ⑤ left subclavian vein, ⑥ right subclavian vein, ⑦ brachiocephalic trunk, ⑧ left brachiocephalic vein, ⑨ right brachiocephalic vein, ⑩ aortic arch, ⑪ superior vena cava, ⑫ pulmonary trunk, ⑬ right atrium, ⑭ left ventricle, sternal plane (red dashed line), aortic valve (blue dashed line).

and the superior heart border joins the upper left and upper right points. The apex beat can be palpated over the left lower border. A laterally displaced apex beat can indicate cardiac enlargement or mediastinal displacement.

Great vessels

The great vessels are the large veins and arteries passing to and from the heart (**Figures 2.17** and **2.18**).

Aorta The ascending aorta arises retrosternally just below the sternal plane and ascends to the right 2nd sternocostal joint where it continues as the arch of the aorta. The arch curves posteriorly and left. It reaches the level of the 1st sternocostal joint where it is seen on radiographs as the aortic knuckle and then continues inferiorly as the descending thoracic aorta at the level of the 2nd left sternocostal joint. The descending aorta passes inferiorly on the left anterolateral side of the upper thoracic vertebrae and moves relatively anterior to the vertebral bodies by T11-T12.

Veins The brachiocephalic veins are formed on both sides by the joining of the internal jugular and subclavian veins posterior to the sternoclavicular joints (**Figures 2.17** and **2.18**). The right and left brachiocephalic veins join posterior to the right 1st costal cartilage to form the superior vena cava, which passes inferiorly to enter the right atrium level with the right 3rd costal cartilage just lateral to the sternum.

Heart valves and auscultation points
The heart valves are located mostly retrosternally (**Figure 2.19**). Heart sounds result from valves closing and pathologies affecting blood flow. Heart sounds tend to travel in the direction of blood flow therefore the auscultation point for a valve differs from its surface marking (**Table 2.4**).

Clinical insight

The heart valves and blood flow through them can be visualised using echocardiography. Depending on the required view the probe can be placed parasternally, apically, subcostally or in the sternal notch.

Sternal angle and plane
The sternal (Louis) angle sits between the sternal body and manubrium at the manubriosternal joint and marks the level of the horizontal sternal plane (**Figure 2.1**). It is palpated as a horizontal ridge ~ 5 cm inferior to the sternal notch. On patients and medical images (**Figure 2.20**), it is a useful marker of the:

- T4–T5 intervertebral disc
- Second costal cartilage (immediately lateral)
- Origin of the aortic arch
- Superior limit of the pulmonary trunk

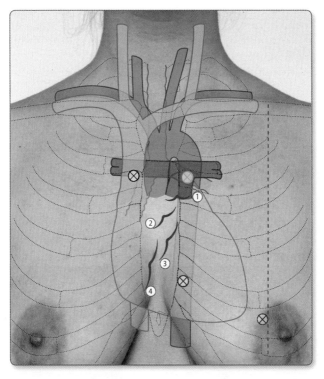

Figure 2.19 Surface markings of the heart valves and auscultation points. ① Pulmonary valve, ② aortic valve, ③ bicuspid (mitral) valve, ④ tricuspid valve, Ⓧ aortic valve auscultation point, Ⓧ pulmonary valve auscultation point, Ⓧ tricuspid valve auscultation point, Ⓧ bicuspid valve auscultation point.

- Pulmonary arteries
- Upper limit of the pericardium
- Tracheal bifurcation and main bronchi
- Horizontal plane separating the superior and inferior mediastinum (**Figure 2.3**)

	Auscultation point	Valve location
Pulmonary valve	2nd left intercostal space just lateral to the sternum	Posterior to the 3rd left costal cartilage and the adjacent sternum
Aortic valve	2nd right intercostal space just lateral to the sternum	Sloping inferiorly and right from 3rd left intercostal space
Bicuspid (mitral) valve	5th left intercostal space midclavicular line (cardiac apex)	Sloping inferiorly and right from the left 4th costal cartilage
Tricuspid valve	4th or 5th left intercostal space just lateral to the sternum	Sloping inferiorly and right from the 4th intercostal space level retrosternally

Table 2.4 Surface markings of the heart valves relative to their auscultation point.

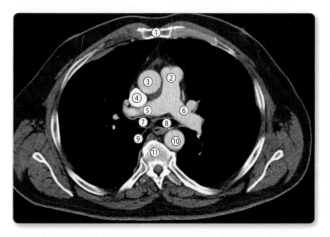

Figure 2.20 Axial CT at the level of the sternal plane/angle. ① Manubriosternal joint, ② pulmonary trunk, ③ ascending aorta, ④ superior vena cava, ⑤ right pulmonary artery, ⑥ left pulmonary artery, ⑦ right main bronchus, ⑧ left main bronchus, ⑨ carina, ⑩ descending aorta, ⑪ lower part of T4 vertebrae.

Abdomen

The abdomen is the inferior part of the trunk, located between the thorax and pelvic cavity. The abdominal cavity is bordered by the inferior surface of the diaphragm, lower part of the thoracic wall, the abdominal wall, pelvic bones, lumbar vertebrae and associated muscle and fascia. Inferiorly the abdominal and pelvic cavities are continuous across the plane of the pelvic inlet. The abdominal cavity contains gastrointestinal and urogenital viscera, and associated vasculature and nerves.

Regions

The abdominal wall is divided into anterolateral and posterior walls by the posterior axillary line. The anterior abdominal wall can be divided into either four or nine regions using standardised intersecting vertical and horizontal reference planes. Such regional models are used for descriptive purposes and help standardise the location of viscera, pathology, procedures and pain.

Function

The abdominal wall serves to retain abdominal viscera, move and support the vertebral column, and to increase intra-abdominal pressure during urination, defecation, vomiting and childbirth. It should be viewed as a functional unit, therefore preservation of innervation and integrity during surgery is important. The wall can distend to accommodate pregnancy, intestinal dilatation, or pathologies such as ascites and pneumoperitoneum. Weakness of the abdominal wall can result in herniation.

Variability

The surface markings stated in this chapter are representative of an average-sized supine patient during quiet breathing. Remember that percussion, palpation, auscultation and ultrasound guidance can be used to further guide surface placement of underlying structures. The surface markings of abdominal viscera may vary depending upon:

- Body position and associated gravity-induced changes
- Organ size and disposition
- Disease states (including thoracic, e.g. hyperinflation)
- Deep inspiration/expiration
- Body mass

3.1 Bony landmarks, joints and ligaments

Margins of the abdominal wall

The superior and inferior osseoligamentous margins of the abdominal wall are easily palpable (**Figure 3.1**).

- The **superior margin** passes from the xiphoid process along the costal margin and along the 12th rib posteriorly
- The **inferior margin** passes from the pubic symphysis (superior part), crest and tubercle, along the inguinal ligament to the anterior superior iliac spine, then posteriorly along the curved iliac crest to the iliolumbar ligament, which connects the iliac crest to the transverse process of the adjacent L4 vertebra

The diaphragm represents the superior limit of the abdominal cavity. It extends superiorly to the level of the 5th costal cartilage in the midclavicular line, and vertebral level T8 (xiphisternal joint) in the midline. The inferior limit is formed by the superior surface of the greater pelvis and associated muscles. Note that the abdominal and pelvic cavities are continuous via the anteroinferiorly sloping plane of the pelvic inlet.

Bony landmarks

Thoracic wall

The lower part of the thoracic wall forms part of the upper abdominal wall. The xiphoid process marks vertebral level T9 and the 7th costal cartilage lies immediately lateral (**Figure 3.2**). The costal margin is the free inferior border of the thoracic cage formed by costal cartilages 7–10. It is palpated inferolaterally from the xiphisternum to rib 10, and is a useful landmark in abdominal examination. Organs such as the liver should not

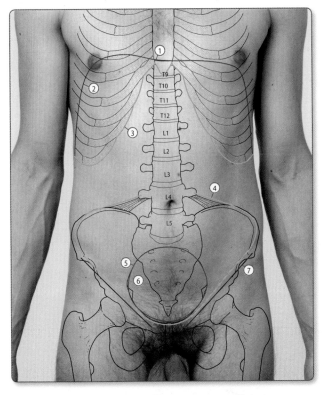

Figure 3.1 Margins of the abdomen. ① Xiphisternal joint, ② diaphragm, ③ superior margin of abdominal wall, ④ inferior margin of abdominal wall, ⑤ plane of pelvic inlet, ⑥ pelvic cavity, ⑦ inguinal ligament.

normally be palpable below the margin. The free ends of the 11th and 12th ribs can be palpated posterolaterally and posteriorly within the muscle of the abdominal wall.

Iliac bone

The iliac bone has several visible and palpable features, which serve as landmarks for vertebral levels and regional borders (**Figure 3.2**).

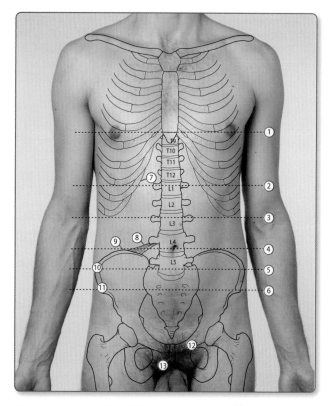

Figure 3.2 Horizontal planes of the thorax and abdomen. ① Xiphisternal plane (T8), ② transpyloric plane (L1), ③ subcostal plane (L3), ④ supracristal plane (L4) (also transumbilical in this subject), ⑤ transtubercular plane (L5), ⑥ interspinous plane (S1), ⑦ costal margin, ⑧ iliolumbar ligament, ⑨ iliac crest (highest point), ⑩ iliac tubercle, ⑪ anterior superior iliac spine, ⑫ pubic tubercle, ⑬ pubic symphysis.

- The **anterior superior iliac spine** is the anteriorly projecting bony prominence located on the anteriormost part of the iliac crest. It marks the attachment of the inguinal ligament and location of the lateral cutaneous nerve of the thigh, which is immediately inferomedial.

- The **posterior superior iliac spine** is a bony prominence located on the posteriormost part of the iliac crest, 3–4 cm from the midvertebral line. The skin over the spine is often indented and referred to as the 'Dimple of Venus'. It marks the level of the S2 spinous process, the lower limit of the subarachnoid space and the sacroiliac joint.
- The **iliac crest** curves posteriorly, superiorly and medially between the anterior superior and posterior superior iliac spines. The highest point of the crest sits posteriorly and marks the supracristal plane (L4), used for landmarking during lumbar puncture.
- The **iliac tubercle** is palpable on the iliac crest around 5–7 cm posterior to the anterior superior iliac spine, and marks the transtubercular plane (L5).

Clinical insight

Femoral hernias normally emerge inferior and lateral to the pubic tubercle whereas inguinal hernias emerge superior to it, and have a variable medial-lateral relationship to the tubercle.

Pubic bone

The raised pubic tubercle is palpable on the superior surface of the pubic bone, about 2–3 cm from the midline (**Figure 3.2**). It marks the medial attachment of the inguinal ligament and serves as a landmark when describing inguinal and femoral hernias. The pubic symphysis is the midline joint between the bodies of the pubic bones.

3.2 Reference planes and regions

Reference planes

A number of horizontal reference planes can be defined each of which marks the level of underlying structures (**Table 3.1, Figure 3.2**).

Regions

The anterior abdominal wall can be divided into four regions (**Figure 3.3**) or nine regions (**Figure 3.4**) by

Clinical insight

Paracentesis of intra-abdominal ascites is performed via needle insertion in the inguinal region, lateral to both the rectus abdominis and inferior epigastric artery.

Plane	Location	Features on plane
Xiphisternal (T8)	Xiphisternal joint	T8 vertebral body; central tendon of diaphragm; diaphragmatic surface of the heart; superior hepatic border
Transpyloric (L1)	Midway between the suprasternal notch and the upper border of the pubic symphysis; passes through tips of the 9th costal cartilages (the distinct change in angle of the costal margin)	L1 Vertebral body; pylorus; duodenum (1st part); attachment of transverse mesocolon; superior mesenteric artery origin; fundus of the gallbladder; portal vein formation; pancreatic neck; kidney hila; renal arteries and veins
Subcostal (L3)	Immediately inferior to the 10th costal cartilage at the lowest anterior point of the costal margin	L3 vertebral body; 3rd part of duodenum; inferior mesenteric artery origin from aorta
Transumbilical (L3–L5/variable)	Umbilicus	Can overlie L3–L4 intervertebral disc, but varies from vertebral body L3-L5
Supracristal (L4)	Highest points of the iliac crests (located posteriorly)	L4 Vertebral body; aortic bifurcation; plane for landmarking L4 spinous process in lumbar puncture
Transtubercular (L5)	Tubercles of the iliac crest (palpable 5–7 cm posterior to the anterior superior iliac spine)	L5 vertebral body; formation of inferior vena cava close to midline
Interspinous (S1)	Anterior superior iliac spines	Termination of small intestine mesentery

Table 3.1 Horizontal planes of the anterior abdominal wall.

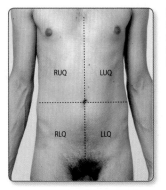

Figure 3.3 Four regions (quadrants) of the anterior abdominal wall. Right upper quadrant (RUQ), left upper quadrant (LUQ), right lower quadrant (RLQ), left lower quadrant (LLQ).

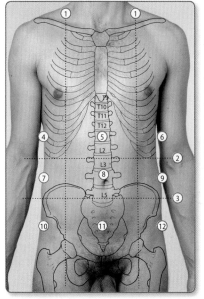

Figure 3.4 Nine regions of the anterior abdominal wall.
① Midclavicular line,
② subcostal plane,
③ transtubercular plane,
④ right hypochondrium,
⑤ epigastrium,
⑥ left hypochondrium,
⑦ right lumbar/flank,
⑧ umbilical,
⑨ left lumbar/flank,
⑩ right inguinal,
⑪ pubic (hypogastrium),
⑫ left inguinal.

	Horizontal planes	Vertical planes
Four-region	Umbilical	Midsternal
Nine-region	Subcostal and transtubercular*	Midclavicular lines (left and right)
*The transpyloric and interspinous planes can be used as alternative horizontal planes in the nine-region model.		

Table 3.2 Reference planes marking the four- and nine-region models of the anterior abdominal wall.

defined vertical and horizontal planes (**Table 3.2**). Regional divisions help standardise descriptions of the location of viscera, pathology, pain and procedures.

3.3 Muscles, tendons and aponeuroses

The majority of the anterolateral abdominal wall is formed by three large flat sheets of muscle passing between the costal margin and pelvic girdle (**Figures 3.5** and **3.6**). The muscles become aponeurotic between the midclavicular line and midline. The transversalis fascia and parietal peritoneum sit deep to the muscles. Knowledge of the muscle layers and direction of their fibres is useful for identification and enabling surgical division whilst minimising damage.

External oblique This is the most superficial muscle. Its fibres pass inferomedially from ribs 5–12 to the linea alba, iliac crest, anterior superior iliac spine and pubic tubercle.

Internal oblique This is located deep to the external oblique. Its lower fibres pass medially and its upper fibres pass superomedially from the thoracolumbar fascia, iliac crest, and lateral inguinal ligament to the linea alba, lower ribs, upper pubis and conjoint tendon.

Transversus abdominis This is the deepest muscle layer. Its fibres pass horizontally from costal cartilages 7–12, the thoracolumbar fascia, iliac crest and inguinal ligament to the linea alba, upper pubis and conjoint tendon.

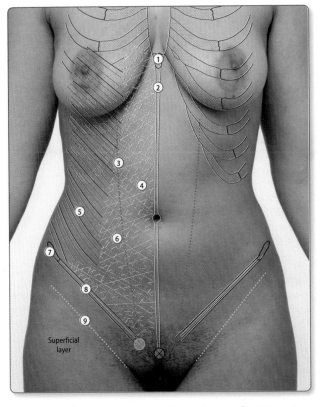

Figure 3.5 Anterior abdominal wall: superficial muscle layer. ① Xiphoid process, ② linea alba, ③ linea semilunaris, ④ rectus sheath, ⑤ external oblique, ⑥ external oblique aponeurosis, ⑦ anterior superior iliac spine, ⑧ inguinal ligament, ⑨ anterior thigh (Holden's) crease, ⊗ pubic tubercle, ⊗ pubic symphysis.

Rectus abdominis This is a paired midline strap muscle passing from costal cartilages 5–7 and the xiphoid to the pubic symphysis and crest. Tendinous intersections give the muscles its characteristic six-pack appearance. Asking a supine patient to raise their head brings the muscle into relief, enabling functional testing.

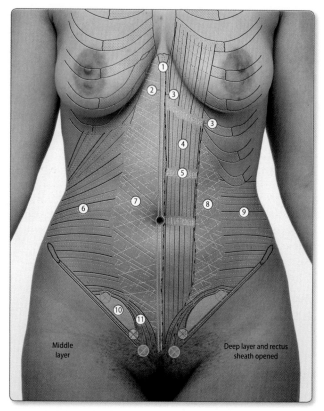

Figure 3.6 Anterior abdominal wall: middle and deep muscle layers.
① Xiphoid process, ② linea alba, ③ cut edges of rectus sheath, ④ rectus abdominis, ⑤ tendinous intersection in rectus abdominis, ⑥ internal oblique, ⑦ internal oblique aponeurosis, ⑧ transversus abdominis aponeurosis, ⑨ transversus abdominis, ⑩ transversalis fascia forming posterior wall of inguinal canal, ⑪ conjoint tendon, Ⓧ position of deep inguinal ring, Ⓧ position of superficial inguinal ring, Ⓧ pubic tubercle.

Conjoint tendon This is formed by the aponeuroses of the internal oblique and transversus abdominis attaching to the pubic bone. It reinforces the tissue behind the superficial inguinal ring therefore weakness can result in direct inguinal hernia formation.

Inguinal ligament This is formed by the aponeurosis of external oblique extending between the anterior superior iliac spine and the pubic tubercle. It sits ~ 2 cm above the anterior thigh crease (Holden's crease). The ligament forms the anterior wall and floor of the inguinal canal and marks the superior border of the femoral triangle.

Linea alba This is the palpable midline raphe/band extending between the xiphoid and pubic symphysis. It is formed by the joining of the aponeuroses of the flat abdominal wall muscles and represents a relatively avascular and aneural plane that is used for surgical access to the abdominal cavity.

> **Clinical insight**
>
> Due to fascial bindings, infections of the anterior abdominal wall can track via fascial planes to the level of the visible anterior thigh crease, which sits ~ 2 cm below the inguinal ligament.

Rectus sheath This encloses the rectus abdominis and the epigastric vessels. It is formed by the aponeuroses of the flat abdominal wall muscles.

Linea semilunaris This is the lateral margin of the rectus abdominis in the rectus sheath and is seen and felt as a curved groove passing from around the 8th costal cartilage to the pubic tubercle.

3.4 Inguinal canal

Location and inguinal rings

The inguinal canal is a passageway through the layers of the lower anterior abdominal wall that runs just above (1–2 cm) the medial half of the inguinal ligament between the deep and superficial inguinal rings (**Figure 3.7**):

- The **deep inguinal ring** is located between the midinguinal point and

> **Clinical insight**
>
> Rectus sheath haematoma results from epigastric vessel bleeding and can cause localised abdominal pain and swelling.

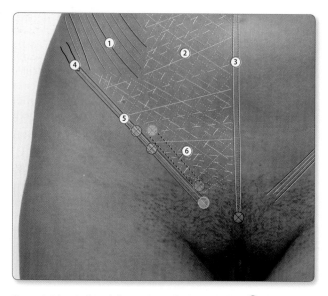

Figure 3.7 Inguinal canal: deep and superficial inguinal rings. (1) External oblique, (2) external oblique aponeurosis, (3) linea alba, (4) anterior superior iliac spine, (5) inguinal ligament, (6) inguinal canal, (X) midpoint of inguinal ligament, (X) position of deep inguinal ring, (X) midinguinal point, (X) position of superficial inguinal ring, (X) pubic tubercle, (X) pubic symphysis.

the midpoint of the inguinal ligament, and 1 cm superior to the inguinal ligament. It is the entrance to the inguinal canal from the abdominal cavity. Indirect inguinal hernias pass into the canal via the deep inguinal ring. Pulsation of the femoral artery can be felt at the midinguinal point (or up to 1.5 cm either side)

- The **superficial inguinal ring** is located immediately superolateral to the pubic tubercle at which point the male spermatic cord is palpable. It represents the exit point from the inguinal canal through the external oblique aponeurosis. The conjoint tendon reinforces it posteriorly (**Figure 3.6**)

The inguinal canal represents a weak spot and area for hernia formation, especially in males. Open inguinal hernia repair is performed via an incision made two finger breadths superior to the anterior thigh crease from the superficial inguinal ring toward the anterior superior iliac spine.

Midinguinal point and midpoint of inguinal ligament

The midinguinal point and the midpoint of the inguinal ligament are reference landmarks used for positioning underlying structures (**Figure 3.7**):

- The **midinguinal point** is situated midway between the anterior superior iliac spine and the midline pubic symphysis. It marks the femoral pulse (± 1.5 cm medial-lateral)
- The **midpoint of the inguinal ligament** is situated midway between the anterior superior iliac spine and the pubic tubercle. The midclavicular line often intersects it

Contents of the inguinal canal

The inguinal canal conveys several structures including:

- The ilioinguinal and genital nerves
- The spermatic cord in the male
- The round ligament of the uterus in the female

Spermatic cord

The spermatic cord can be palpated as a collection of soft fibres/cords passing inferiorly from the superficial inguinal ring to the superior pole of the testicle (**Figures 3.8** and **6.20**). The cord contains:

- The ductus deferens
- The testicular, deferential and cremasteric arteries and veins
- The genital, ilioinguinal and sympathetic nerves

The cord is covered by three layers, which are extensions of the external oblique aponeurosis (external spermatic fascia), internal oblique fascia (cremasteric fascia) and the transversalis fascia (internal spermatic fascia). Indirect inguinal hernias pass through the inguinal canal and are therefore covered by the

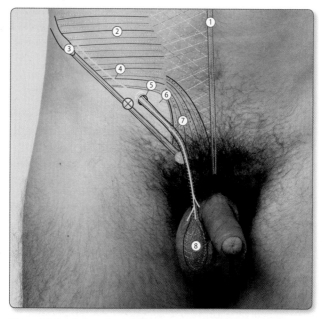

Figure 3.8 Inguinal canal: view of the spermatic cord with the external oblique muscle removed. (1) Linea alba, (2) internal oblique, (3) anterior superior iliac spine, (4) ilioinguinal nerve, (5) deep inguinal ring, (6) transversalis fascia, (7) spermatic cord, (8) testicle, (X) midpoint of inguinal ligament, (X) pubic tubercle.

layers of the cord. Knowledge of the cord's position, structure and contents are important for vasectomy and examination. For example, varicocele of the testicular vein (pampiniform plexus) causes an irregular cord swelling.

3.5 Neurovasculature and lymphatics

Dermatomes
The abdominal dermatomes curve anteroinferiorly around the abdominal wall from the midvertebral to the midsternal

line (**Figure 1.38**). Superiorly thoracic spinal nerves emerge at the costal margin onto the anterior abdominal where they are at risk during surgical incision. Adjacent dermatomes overlap considerably. Three landmark dermatomes can be identified on the anterior abdomen:

- T6 at the xiphisternum
- T10 at the umbilicus
- L1 below the inguinal ligament

Intra-abdominal vasculature

The main vessels of the abdominal cavity run close to the midline then pass around the pelvic brim to the lower limb (**Figures 3.9** and **3.17**).

Abdominal aorta and branches

The abdominal aorta passes through the diaphragm at T12 and runs along, or just left of, the median plane where its pulsations can normally be palpated in the supine patient, especially if lean. Abdominal aortic aneurysms (AAAs) can be felt along this line. Knowledge of the locations of the main branches of the aorta is useful for vessel sonography, auscultation and for locating the closely associated autonomic nerve plexi, which innervate the gut tube and pelvic viscera. The plexi can be anaesthetised under radiographic guidance in cases of persistent severe pain.

Anterior branches There are three main anterior branches with associated autonomic plexi (**Table 3.3**).

Lateral branches The renal arteries arise laterally at L1 on the transpyloric plane on either side of the midline. The vessels can be examined via ultrasound or auscultated for bruits associated with stenosis.

Terminal branches The aorta bifurcates into common iliac vessels at vertebral level L4 (supracristal plane). The iliac vessels can be auscultated on the transtubercular plane either side of the midline.

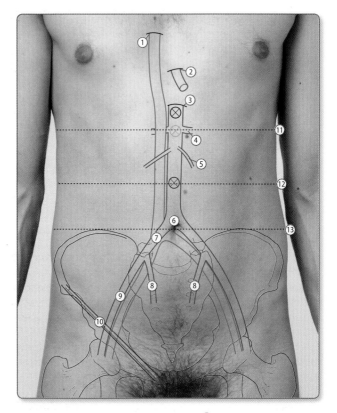

Figure 3.9 Vasculature of the abdominal cavity. ① Inferior vena cava (T8), ② oesophagus (T10), ③ abdominal aorta (T12), ④ renal artery, ⑤ gonadal artery, ⑥ abdominal aorta bifurcation (L4), ⑦ common iliac artery and vein, ⑧ internal iliac artery and vein, ⑨ external iliac artery and vein, ⑩ inguinal ligament, ⑪ transpyloric plane (L1), ⑫ subcostal plane (L3), ⑬ supracristal plane (L4), Ⓧ coeliac trunk origin point, Ⓧ superior mesenteric artery origin point, Ⓧ inferior mesenteric artery origin point.

Veins

The inferior vena cava is formed just right of the midline by the joining of the common iliac veins at L5 (transtubercular plane). It runs to the right of the aorta and median plane, passes through

Artery and plexus	Vertebral level and plane of origin	Region supplied/ innervated
Coeliac	T12 (2 cm above transpyloric plane)	Foregut
Superior mesenteric	L1 (transpyloric plane)	Midgut
Inferior mesenteric	L3 (subcostal plane)	Hindgut

Table 3.3 Level of origin of the midline aortic branches and their associated autonomic plexi.

the diaphragm at T8 (plane of xiphisternal joint) to immediately enter the right atrium. The renal veins join the inferior vena cava at L1 (transpyloric plane).

Neurovasculature of the abdominal wall

Abdominal wall neurovasculature travel together, curving anteroinferiorly toward the anterior midline (midsternal line) (**Figure 3.10**). In general the thoracoabdominal nerves and arteries continue onto the abdominal wall along the same inclination as the rib to which they were associated, and become more horizontal as they approach the midline. The main neurovascular plane of the abdominal wall sits between the internal oblique and transversus abdominis. Nerves and vessels then pierce the rectus abdominis to supply it and overlying tissues.

Nerves can be damaged during surgery or endoscopic trochar placement (**Table 3.4**). Nerve damage can lead to chronic pain and/or to abdominal wall muscle paralysis and consequent predisposition to hernia formation.

Arteries of the abdominal wall

The subcostal and lumbar arteries curve anteroinferiorly around the abdominal wall from the descending aorta toward the anterior midline. The remaining vessels follow atypical patterns (**Figure 3.10**):

- **Superior epigastric artery** passes inferiorly within the rectus sheath, lateral to the midline and deep to rectus abdominis

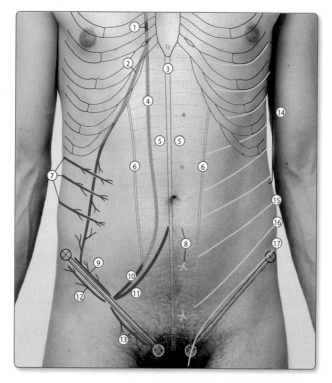

Figure 3.10 Anterior abdominal wall: neurovasculature. ① Internal thoracic artery, ② musculophrenic artery, ③ linea alba, ④ superior epigastric artery, ⑤ rectus sheath, ⑥ linea semilunaris, ⑦ intercostal/subcostal/lumbar arteries, ⑧ anterior cutaneous nerve branches, ⑨ deep circumflex iliac artery, ⑩ inferior epigastric artery, ⑪ superficial epigastric artery, ⑫ superficial circumflex iliac artery, ⑬ superficial and deep external pudendal arteries, ⑭ intercostal nerves (T6–T11), ⑮ subcostal nerve (T12), ⑯ iliohypogastric nerve (L1), ⑰ ilioinguinal nerve (L1), Ⓧ anterior superior iliac spine, Ⓧ pubic tubercle.

- **Inferior epigastric artery** passes superomedially from the midinguinal point (± 1.5cm medial-lateral) and into the lower rectus sheath, which it ascends deep to rectus abdominis and lateral to the midline

Nerve(s) at risk of damage	Root value	Procedure/incision (Figure 3.1)
Thoracoabdominal	T6–T11	Cholecystectomy via a subcostal (Kocher) incision
Subcostal	T12	Renal surgery via a dorsal lumbotomy incision
Iliohypogastric	L1	Appendectomy via a transverse skin crease incision at McBurney point
Ilioinguinal	L1	Cesarean section via suprapubic incision; inguinal canal incision

Table 3.4 Abdominal wall nerves at risk of damage during surgical procedures/ incisions.

- **Musculophrenic artery** passes inferolaterally along the costal margin then inferiorly from the 10th costal cartilage toward the anterior superior iliac spine
- **Superficial epigastric artery** passes superomedially from the midinguinal point ($\pm$ 1.5 cm) toward the umbilicus
- **Circumflex iliac arteries** (superficial and deep) pass superolaterally from the midinguinal point ($\pm$ 1.5 cm) towards the anterior superior iliac spine in superficial or deep tissues
- **External pudendal arteries** (superficial and deep) pass inferomedially from the midinguinal point ($\pm$ 1.5 cm) toward the mons pubis in superficial or deep tissues

Lymphatic drainage

Lymphatics from the anterolateral abdominal wall above the umbilicus drain to axillary and parasternal nodes and those from regions below the umbilicus to superficial inguinal nodes.

3.6 Surgical incisions of the abdominal wall

The choice and size of surgical incision is based upon the structure to be accessed, the anticipated pathology and the required surgical field (**Figure 3.11**). Attention needs to be paid to the location and direction of travel of abdominal wall neurovasculature to minimise damage and functional loss.

- A **vertical midline incision** passes vertically through the linea alba enabling quick entry to the peritoneum. The linea alba provides an aneural and relatively avascular plane
- A **paramedian incision** runs parallel to the linea alba and pass through the rectus sheath. The epigastric vessels can be identified and preserved, and the rectus abdominis divided or displaced laterally toward its nerve supply

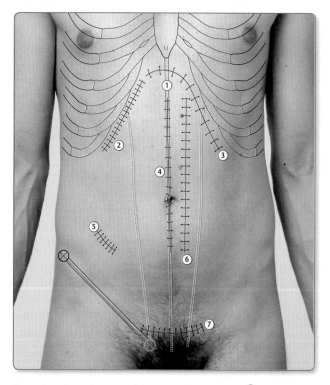

Figure 3.11 Surgical incisions of the anterior abdominal wall. ① Line alba, ② subcostal (Kocher) incision, ③ extension of subcostal incision (double Kocher/roof top), ④ vertical midline incision, ⑤ transverse skin crease incision at McBurney's point, ⑥ paramedian incision, ⑦ suprapubic (Pfannenstiel) incision, ⓧ anterior superior iliac spine, ⓧ pubic tubercle.

- A **subcostal (Kocher) incision** parallels the costal margin (two finger breadths below) from just lateral to the linea alba. The T9 nerve must be identified and preserved. The superior epigastric artery and the thoracoabdominal nerves are at risk. A double Kocher (roof top) incision provides access to gastric and diaphragmatic structures
- A **suprapubic (Pfannenstiel) incision** runs transversely 5 cm above the pubic symphysis and is used to access pelvic organs or for cesarean delivery. Risks damage to the ilioiguinal nerve
- A **transverse skin crease incision** at McBurney's point (one third of the way up a line joining the anterior superior iliac spine to the umbilicus) provides access to the caecum and appendix. The abdominal wall muscles are split and separated and the transversalis fascia and peritoneum cut. There is a risk of damage to the iliohypogastric and ilioinguinal nerves with associated risk of hernia formation

3.7 Viscera

Regional contents

Four-region model

A knowledge of the regional location of the viscera is essential for effective clinical examination and procedures. The position of abdominal viscera can be described in relation to the four-region model (**Table 3.5**).

Nine-region model

Localisation of viscera using the nine-region model is not as reliable as with the four-region model since many viscera sit across boundaries. Common sites for viscera distribution are as follows:

- The **epigastric region** contains the stomach, liver, gallbladder, transverse colon, lesser sac, abdominal aorta, duodenum pancreas, kidneys, suprarenal glands and both the origin and plexus of the coeliac trunk and superior mesenteric artery
- The **umbilical region** contains small intestine, root of the mesentery, the abdominal aorta and inferior mesenteric artery origin and plexus

Right upper quadrant	Left upper quadrant
Colon (ascending, hepatic flexure); duodenum (parts 1–3); gallbladder; biliary tree; inferior vena cava; pancreas (head and neck); pylorus; right kidney; ureter and suprarenal gland	Colon (splenic flexure and descending); duodenum (part 4); left kidney; ureter and suprarenal gland; pancreas (body and tail); spleen; stomach; jejunum and ileum
Right lower quadrant	**Left lower quadrant**
Colon (caecum, appendix and ascending); inferior vena cava; right ductus deferens; ovary; uterine tube; ureter and ileum	Colon (descending and sigmoid); left ductus deferens; ovary; uterine tube; ureter, jejunum and ileum

Table 3.5 Visceral contents of each of the four abdominal regions (quadrants).

- The **pubic region** contains the small intestine, sigmoid colon, upper rectum, ovary, uterine tube, distended bladder, enlarged uterus, and common iliac arteries
- The **left and right hypochondriac regions** contain the diaphragm and costodiaphragmatic recesses. The left also contains the stomach, spleen, pancreatic tail and splenic flexure of the colon and the right also contains the liver and the hepatic flexure of the colon
- The **lumbar (loin, flank or lateral) regions** contain the ascending (right) and descending (left) colons, respectively, and the small intestine
- The **inguinal regions** (also known as the iliac fossa) contain the caecum and appendix (right) and the sigmoid colon (left)

Localisation of regional pain

The location of pain is often described using the nine-region model. This provides clues as to possible differential diagnoses.

> **Clinical insight**
>
> The bladder can be catheterised via a suprapubic approach. The catheter is passed through the anterior abdominal wall but not through the peritoneum.

True visceral pain from the gut tube (foregut, midgut or hindgut) often refers to the three midline regions, respectively. Organ-specific pain can also be felt in the region occupied by the organ (**Table 3.6**).

R. Hypochondrium	Epigastrium	L. Hypochondrium
Liver abscess; hepatitis; gall bladder/biliary tree; cholecystitis; cholelithiasis	Foregut pain; aortic aneurysm; pancreatitis; ulcer; gastritis; reflux; myocardial infarction; pericarditis	Constipation; splenic infarct; abscess; colitis; diverticulitis; pyelonephritis
R. lumbar/flank	**Umbilical**	**L. lumbar/flank**
Ascending colitis; nephrolithiasis; pyelonephritis	Midgut pain; enteritis; intestinal obstruction; mesenteric occlusion	Descending colitis; nephrolithiasis; pyelonephritis
R. inguinal	**Pubic**	**L. inguinal**
Appendicitis; gonadal pathology; gastroenteritis; inguinal hernia	Hindgut pain; uterine pathology; urinary tract infection/obstruction; endometriosis; pelvic inflammatory disease	Diverticulitis; colitis; gonadal pathology; inguinal hernia; ulcerative colitis

Table 3.6 Regional localisation/referral of pain due to visceral pathology, based on the nine-region model.

Liver and gallbladder

Liver This is located under the diaphragm, mainly in the right hypochondrium and epigastrium (**Figures 3.12** and **3.13**). The left lobe extends into the left hypochondrium. It can be mapped out between three points (**Table 3.7**).

The lower border of the liver follows the right costal margin and is not normally palpable below it. However, it can be palpable in liver disease or metastasis. In some the liver drops below the costal margin near the midline, and the right lobe can extend into the right lumbar region. The liver's presence in the right hypochondrium pushes the right diaphragmatic dome superiorly and results in an inferior movement of the liver on inspiration.

> **Clinical insight**
>
> Irritation of the diaphragm via local abdominal pathology, free fluid or gas can produce shoulder pain due to referral via the phrenic nerve (C3–5).

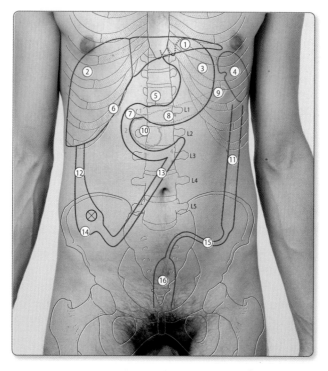

Figure 3.12 Abdominal viscera and mesentery attachments. ① Left lobe of liver overlying fundus of stomach, ② right lobe of liver, ③ stomach, ④ spleen, ⑤ pylorus, ⑥ gallbladder fundus (9th costal cartilage tip), ⑦ duodenum (four parts labelled 1–4), ⑧ neck and body of pancreas, ⑨ tail of pancreas, ⑩ head of pancreas, ⑪ site of descending colon, ⑫ site of ascending colon, ⑬ attachment (root) of small intestine mesentery, ⑭ site of caecum, ⑮ attachment of sigmoid colon mesentery, ⑯ site of rectum, Ⓧ site of appendix attachment to caecum.

Clinical insight

The anterior, lateral and posterior liver surfaces are surrounded by the costodiaphragmatic recess, therefore pneumothorax is a risk following percutaneous needle biopsy.

Gallbladder This is located inferior to the liver with its fundus situated close to the tip of the 9th right costal cartilage. Pressure under the right costal margin at the 9th

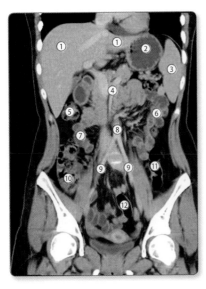

Figure 3.13 Coronal CT of the abdomen: viscera and arteries. ① Liver, ② stomach (fundus), ③ spleen, ④ superior mesenteric artery, ⑤ hepatic flexure of colon, ⑥ jejunum, ⑦ ileum, ⑧ abdominal aorta, ⑨ common iliac arteries, ⑩ caecum, ⑪ descending colon, ⑫ sigmoid colon.

Point	Surface location
Left upper	5th rib in the midclavicular line
Right upper	5th rib in the midclavicular line
Right lower	10th right costal cartilage

Table 3.7 Surface marking of the liver relative to the thoracic wall when viewed anteriorly.

costal cartilage level followed by inspiration can elicit pain in cholecystitis (Murphy sign).

Stomach, duodenum and pancreas

Stomach This is variable in size and position. It is located mainly in the epigastrium and left hypochondrium (**Figure 3.12**). The gastric fundus sits under the diaphragm level with the left 5th rib in the midclavicular line and when erect accumulates gas, which is visible on radiographs. The pylorus sits on the transpyloric plane just right of the midline. Palpation of the epigastric region can reveal gastric tumours and auscultation of the stomach can reveal an audible succussion splash associated with intestinal obstruction.

Duodenum This is continuous with the gastric pylorus on the transpyloric plane. The duodenum is C-shaped and has four parts:
- The 1st part passes right along the transpyloric plane toward the right 9th costal cartilage
- The 2nd part passes inferiorly to the subcostal plane
- The 3rd part passes left along the subcostal plane to a point just left of the midline
- The 4th part passes superiorly and anteriorly to meet the jejunum at the root of the mesentery, just left of L2

Pancreas This sits on the posterior abdominal wall. The pancreatic head and uncinate process sit in the C-shaped curve of the duodenum to the right of the midline between the subcostal and transpyloric planes. The pancreatic neck passes leftwards across the midline on the transpyloric plane (L1). The pancreatic tail extends into the left hypochondrium toward the spleen.

Spleen

The spleen is located in the posterolateral part of the left hypochondrium deep to ribs 9–11, the diaphragm and the costodiaphragmatic recess (**Figures 3.12–3.14**). An enlarged spleen projects from the left costal margin towards the right iliac fossa. Rib trauma can damage both the spleen and parietal pleura resulting in pneumo- or haemothorax.

Small intestine and root of mesentery

The small intestine, consisting of the jejunum and ileum, is located mainly in the umbilical and pubic regions, , but extends bilaterally into the lumbar and inguinal regions (**Figures 3.13** and **3.14**). The mesentery of the small intestine attaches via a root to the posterior abdominal wall (**Figure 3.12**). The root passes inferiorly and rightwards from a point just left of the

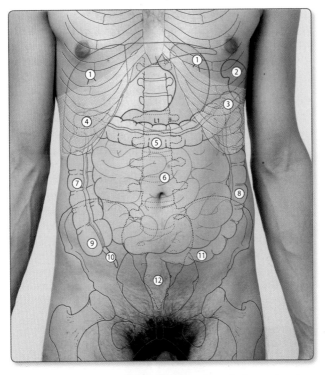

Figure 3.14 Small and large intestine. ① Region of costodiaphragmatic recess (white hatch), ② spleen, ③ splenic flexure of colon, ④ hepatic flexure of colon, ⑤ transverse colon, ⑥ small intestine (ileum and jejunum), ⑦ ascending colon, ⑧ descending colon, ⑨ caecum, ⑩ appendix, ⑪ sigmoid colon, ⑫ rectum.

L2 vertebral body (2 cm below the transpyloric plane) to a point anterior to the right sacroiliac joint (on the interspinous plane).

Caecum and appendix

The caecum connects with the ileum at the ileocaecal junction in the right iliac fossa. The appendix normally originates from the posterior surface of the caecum, the surface marking of the which is approximated by the McBurney point; one third of the way up a line drawn from the anterior superior iliac spine to the umbilicus. The position of the appendix is variable ranging from retrocaecal to projection into the pelvic cavity.

Colon and mesocolon

The ascending colon passes superiorly from the caecum, in the right iliac fossa, through the right lumbar region to the right hypochondrium, where it contacts the liver and turns left at the hepatic flexure to continue as the transverse colon (**Figure 3.14**). The transverse colon travels across to the left hypochondrium, where it contacts the spleen at the splenic flexure and turns downwards to continue as the descending colon. The transverse colon can droop into the umbilical, or pubic, regions (**Figure 3.15**).

The transverse mesocolon (transverse colon mesentery) attaches to the posterior abdominal wall along the transpyloric plane. The descending colon passes inferiorly to the right iliac

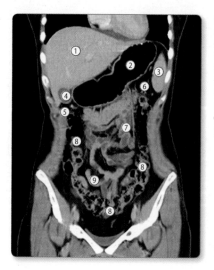

Figure 3.15 Coronal CT of the abdomen: small and large intestine. (1) Liver, (2) stomach, (3) spleen, (4) gallbladder, (5) hepatic flexure of colon, (6) splenic flexure of colon, (7) jejunum, (8) transverse colon (low lying), (9) ileum.

fossa, where it is continuous with the sigmoid colon, which joins the rectum at S3 near the midline.

Kidney, ureter and renal angle

Kidneys These are located on the posterior abdominal wall, either side of the midline (**Figures 3.16** and **3.17**). Each kidney extends between T11 and L2/3 with

Clinical insight

Stool can be palpated as a firm impressionable mass in the descending/ sigmoid colon, especially during constipation.

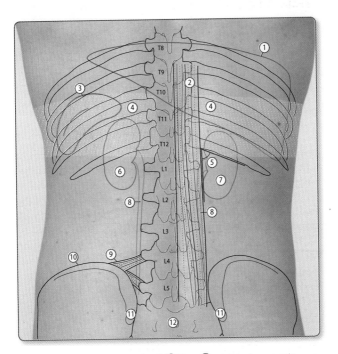

Figure 3.16 Posterior abdominal wall. ① Liver, ② erector spinae muscle group, ③ spleen, ④ region of costodiaphragmatic recess (white hatch), ⑤ renal angle. ⑥ left kidney, ⑦ right kidney, ⑧ ureter, ⑨ iliolumbar ligament, ⑩ iliac crest, ⑪ posterior superior iliac spine, ⑫ sacrum.

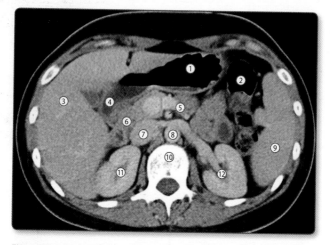

Figure 3.17 Axial CT of the abdomen: transpyloric plane and kidney.
① Stomach, ② transverse colon, ③ liver, ④ duodenum 1st part, ⑤ superior
mesenteric artery, ⑥ pancreas, ⑦ inferior vena cava, ⑧ aorta, ⑨ spleen,
⑩ lower part of L1 vertebra, ⑪ right kidney, ⑫ left kidney and hilum.

the hilum located at L1 (transpyloric plane). The posterior
surface of the kidney overlies the diaphragm and costodiaphragmatic recess. The ureters pass from the renal pelvis at
L1, inferiorly along the tips of the transverse processes of the
lumbar vertebrae, which are a useful radiographic landmark
when looking for ureteric calculi.

The kidney can be palpated in the renal angle, a region
located between the lower border of rib 12 and the lateral
border of the paravertebral muscles. Healthy kidneys are not
normally palpable.

Upper limb

The upper limb is formed by the arm, forearm and hand. It articulates proximally with the pectoral girdle at the shoulder joint. The pectoral girdle, formed by the scapula, clavicle and associated muscles, acts as a mobile articulation with the outer surface of the thoracic wall and sternum. Within the forearm the terms medial and lateral are synonymous with ulnar and radial, respectively.

Compartments

Strong deep fascia surrounds the limb and joins with bone via intermuscular septa, thus forming compartments (**Table 4.1**). The septa can provide surgical planes to the underlying bones. Increases in intracompartmental pressure (compartment syndrome) due to bleeds or infection are characterised by limb pain and varying levels of pallor, pulselessness, paraesthesia and paralysis.

4.1 Pectoral girdle, shoulder and arm

Bones, joints and ligaments

Scapula

The scapula sits over the upper posterior and lateral thoracic walls between the T2–T7 spinous processes (**Figures 4.1** and **4.2**). Several of its borders and features are palpable.

- The **coracoid process** is the bony prominence palpable through muscle ~ 2 cm inferior to the lateral clavicle. Impingement of the process against the humeral lesser tuberosity can produce regional tenderness
- The **acromion** is the shelf of bone located superior to the shoulder and lateral to the coracoid. It meets the scapula spine posteriorly at the distinct acromial angle
- The **spine**, a superolaterally inclined bony ridge, is located on the posterior of the scapula. Medially the spine marks the T3 spinous process

Region	Fascia	Compartments and septa surface marking
Arm	Brachial	Anterior and posterior; septa sit in the grooves between biceps and triceps
Forearm	Antebrachial	Anterior and posterior; septa sit on the posterior border of ulna and medial border of brachioradialis

Table 4.1 Fascia and compartments of the upper limb.

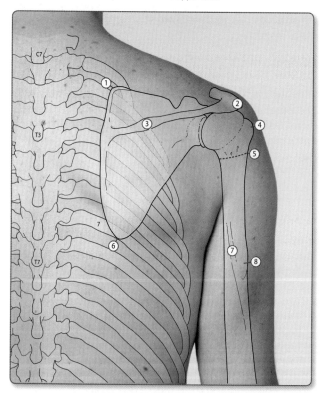

Figure 4.1 Posterior view of pectoral girdle, shoulder and arm. ① Superior angle, ② angle of the acromion, ③ deltoid tubercle of scapula spine, ④ greater tubercle, ⑤ surgical neck of humerus, ⑥ inferior angle, ⑦ spiral groove of humerus, ⑧ deltoid tuberosity.

- The **deltoid tubercle** is the bony prominence on the medial part of the spine that marks the medial limit of the deltoid attachment
- The **inferior angle** is palpable and visible. The triangle of auscultation sits medially (**Figure 4.5** and Chapter 7)

Humerus

Several parts of the proximal humerus can be identified via deep palpation (**Figure 4.2**). The humeral head is not normally palpable, however it becomes palpable inferomedial to the acromion following anterior shoulder dislocation.

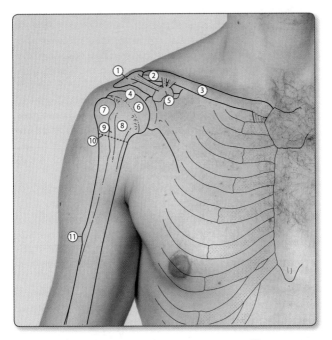

Figure 4.2 Anterior view of pectoral girdle, shoulder and arm. ① Acromion, ② acromioclavicular joint, ③ clavicle, ④ anatomical neck of humerus, ⑤ coracoid process, ⑥ articular head, ⑦ greater tubercle, ⑧ lesser tubercle, ⑨ intertubercular groove, ⑩ surgical neck, ⑪ deltoid tubercle.

- The **surgical neck** sits ~ 5 cm inferior to the acromion. It marks the level of the axillary nerve and circumflex humeral vessels, which must be avoided during shoulder surgery and intramuscular deltoid injection
- The **spiral groove** runs inferolaterally around the posterior shaft and marks the position of the radial nerve and profunda brachii artery. It is ~ 6.5 cm in length (centred on the deltoid tuberosity) starting medially ~ 17–20 cm proximal to the medial epicondyle and ending laterally ~ 11–13 cm proximal to the lateral epicondyle
- The **lesser tubercle** is located on the anteromedial surface of the proximal humerus. It is palpable lateral to the coracoid process, through deltoid
- The **intertubercular sulcus/bicipital groove** runs vertically and sits inferior to the anterolateral border of the acromion. Palpation of the lesser tubercle followed by medial shoulder rotation aids identification. Regional pain/tenderness indicates bicipital tendonitis. The injection site for the groove is ~ 2–3 cm inferior to the anterolateral acromial border
- The **greater tubercle** is the most lateral bony prominence of the proximal humerus, palpable inferolateral to the acromion. Regional tenderness can indicate rotator cuff injury

Clavicle

The lateral one third of the clavicle is flattened whereas the medial two thirds are rounded. It joins the manubrium medially (**Chapter 2**) and the acromion laterally. The acromioclavicular joint can dislocate or become inflamed. Joint injection is via either a superior or anterior approach. The joint is palpated as a sagittal ridge ~ 2–3 cm medial to the lateral acromion and the joint space is opened via lateral shoulder rotation.

> ## Clinical insight
>
> Fractures affect the regions of the clavicle in the following order: middle third > lateral third > medial third.

Shoulder joint

The shoulder joint space sits inferior to the acromion and coracoacromial ligament and extends to a point ~ 3 cm inferior to the coracoid process, which itself sits over the joint (**Figures 4.3** and **4.4**). Knowledge of joint space location enables arthrocentesis or injection. A needle can either be inserted below the palpable coracoid process and directed superolaterally or inserted 2 cm inferomedial to the acromial angle and directed toward the coracoid process.

Ligaments

Several strong ligaments join the clavicle to the scapula (**Figure 4.3**). Some can be identified via deep palpation between the attachment points and are subject to injury or rupture following trauma/excess wear:

- The **costoclavicular ligament** joins the medial clavicle to the first costal cartilage. It should be avoided when cannulating the subclavian vein
- The **coracoclavicular ligament** (consisting of trapezoid and conoid parts) joins the coracoid process to the inferior clavicle. Rupture often accompanies acromioclavicular joint dislocation

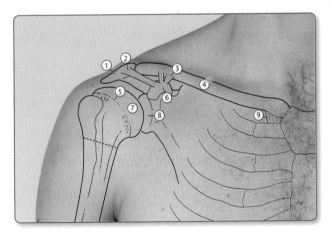

Figure 4.3 Shoulder joint and anterior pectoral girdle ligaments. ① Acromion, ② coracoacromial ligament, ③ coracoclavicular ligament, ④ clavicle, ⑤ anatomical neck of humerus, ⑥ coracoid process, ⑦ humeral head, ⑧ glenoid fossa, ⑨ costoclavicular ligament.

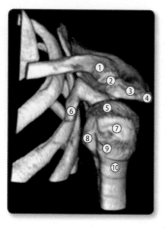

Figure 4.4 3D rendered CT image of the anterior shoulder. ① Clavicle, ② acromioclavicular joint, ③ acromion, ④ acromial angle, ⑤ humeral head, ⑥ coracoid process, ⑦ greater tubercle, ⑧ lesser tubercle, ⑨ intertubercular groove, ⑩ surgical neck.

- The **coracoacromial ligament** joins the coracoid with the acromion collectively forming the coracoacromial arch. The arch is palpable through deltoid and represents a point for impingement or wear of supraspinatus and the subacromial bursa

Muscles, tendons and regions
Shoulder muscles

Rotator cuff muscles These support the shoulder joint. The cuff is formed by four muscles passing between the scapula and proximal humerus (**Figure 4.5**). The muscles are often injured therefore knowledge of their location and points of wear helps when diagnosing the causes of shoulder pain.

- **Supraspinatus** sits above the scapula spine and passes under the coracoacromial arch to the superior surface of the greater tuberosity. It is the most commonly injured cuff muscle
- **Infraspinatus** sits below the scapula spine and passes to the posterosuperior surface of the greater tubercle
- **Teres minor** passes from the lateral border or the scapula to the posteroinferior surface of the greater tubercle
- **Subscapularis** originates from the anterior scapula and is therefore only palpable at its attachment to the lesser tubercle

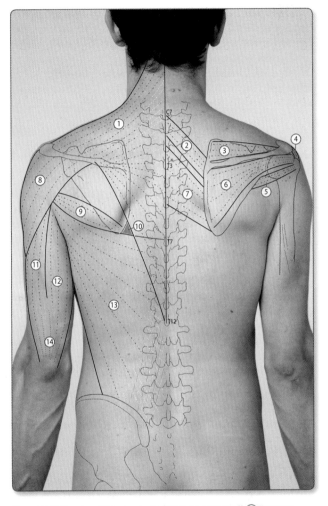

Figure 4.5 Muscles of the scapula, shoulder and rotator cuff. ① Trapezius, ② rhomboid minor, ③ supraspinatus, ④ supraspinatus tendon, ⑤ teres minor, ⑥ infraspinatus, ⑦ rhomboid major, ⑧ deltoid, ⑨ teres major, ⑩ triangle of auscultation (orange), ⑪ triceps lateral head, ⑫ triceps long head, ⑬ latissimus dorsi, ⑭ triceps tendon.

Supraspinatus is separated from the coracoacromial arch by the subacromial bursa. Both are susceptible to impingement and wear resulting in shoulder pain that is exacerbated via palpation in the acromiohumeral sulcus. Bursitis can be treated via steroid injection. The needle is inserted ~ 2 cm inferior to the midpoint of the lateral acromion and directed anteromedially following the slope of the acromion by ~ 3–5 cm.

Teres major This can be felt passing superolaterally from the inferior angle and lateral border of the scapula toward the axilla. It forms part of the posterior axillary fold.

Deltoid This attaches to the scapula spine, acromion and lateral clavicle, its fibres converge on the deltoid tuberosity halfway down the lateral humerus. It covers the shoulder and contributes to its rounded contour, which is lost following dislocation or axillary nerve injury.

Superficial extrinsic layer of the back
Trapezius This is a large flat triangular-shaped muscle of the back and neck. It passes from the posterior cranium, nuchal ligament, and thoracic vertebral spines, to the scapula spine, acromion and lateral third of the clavicle. Its free upper border is seen and palpated passing inferolaterally in the posterior neck.

Latissimus dorsi This is a large flat superficial muscle of the back that attaches to the lower six thoracic vertebrae, lower ribs, thoracolumbar fascia and iliac crest and passes to the lesser tubercle of the humerus. Its lateral border forms the posterior axillary fold (**Chapter 2**) and can be traced inferiorly to the iliac crest.

Rhomboid minor and major These are located deep to trapezius, and pass from the spinous processes of C7–T1 (minor) and T2–T5 (major) to the medial scapula border. Scapula retraction enables palpation of the contracted rhomboids.

Arm muscles

Triceps brachii This is located posteriorly (**Figure 4.5**). Its lateral head sits in the upper lateral arm and its long head in the upper medial arm. Both pass deep to deltoid. Its medial head attaches to the posterior humeral shaft. All three heads converge distally on the broad triceps tendon, which attaches to the ulnar olecranon and is palpable. Tapping the tendon tests the C7–8 reflex.

Biceps brachii This forms the prominent rounded muscle belly of the anterior arm (**Figure 4.6**). Its short head arises from the coracoid process and its long head tendon passes through the intertubercular groove where it can become worn and painfully inflamed. Subsequent tendon rupture causes a gathering of the muscle in the distal arm (Popeye deformity). Distally the biceps tendon and aponeurosis pass through the cubital fossa. Tapping the tendon tests the C5–6 reflex.

Infraclavicular fossa/deltopectoral triangle This is the depression located between the clavicular attachments of deltoid and pectoralis major, below the junction of the lateral and middle thirds of the clavicle. The region marks:

- The superior part of the deltopectoral groove
- The location of deltopectoral lymph nodes and cephalic vein
- An entry site for subclavian vein cannulation (central line)

Neurovasculature

Nerves

Brachial plexus and branches The brachial plexus (C5–T1) innervates the upper limb and pectoral girdle. The plexus passes through the neck posterior to the subclavian artery (**see Chapter 8**) then wraps itself around the axillary artery (with which it can be landmarked) to enter the limb. Its main branches arise in the axilla (**Table 4.2** and **Figure 4.7**).

Arteries

The subclavian artery and its branches supply the upper limb (**Figure 4.7**). Knowledge of vessel location enables peripheral

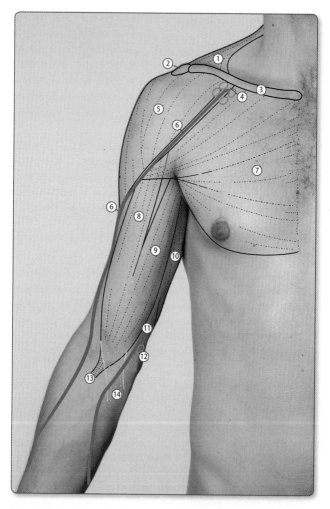

Figure 4.6 Anterior pectoral girdle and arm muscles. ① Trapezius, ②
acromion, ③ clavicle, ④ infraclavicular fossa containing deltopectoral lymph
nodes and cephalic vein, ⑤ deltoid, ⑥ cephalic vein, ⑦ pectoralis major,
⑧ biceps long head, ⑨ biceps short head, ⑩ triceps long head, ⑪ basilic
vein, ⑫ cubital lymph nodes, ⑬ biceps tendon, ⑭ biceps aponeurosis.

Nerve	Surface marking/route
Median	Accompanies the brachial artery through the arm, sitting lateral to it proximally and medial to it distally
Radial	Passes around the humeral spiral groove with which it is landmarked and enters the anterior arm two thirds of the way down a line from acromial angle to the lateral epicondyle
Ulnar	Passes distally along the medial arm, posterior to the brachial artery and anterior to triceps. Distally it passes posterior to the medial epicondyle where it can be palpated as a firm cord or injured. It can be anaesthetised 2 cm proximal to groove between the medial epicondyle and the olecranon
Axillary	Passes around the posterior aspect of the humeral surgical neck ~ 5 cm inferior to the acromion. It should be landmarked and avoided during intramuscular injection and lateral approaches to the shoulder
Musculocutaneous	Passes inferiorly deep to biceps brachii to emerge from its lateral border ~ 2 cm proximal to the elbow. Needs to be identified during an anterior surgical approach to the humerus

Table 4.2 Main branches of the brachial plexus in the arm.

pulse examination, arterial blood sampling, the landmarking of closely associated nerves and helps limit injury during surgical access and venous cannulation.

- The **subclavian artery** curves superolaterally from behind the sternoclavicular joint and passes posterior to the medial third of the clavicle. Its pulsations are palpable in the supra-clavicular triangle lateral to sternocleidomastoid where it is at risk of damage during subclavian vein cannulation
- The **axillary artery** curves through the axilla from the mid-clavicle to the region behind the intersection of pectoralis major and biceps short head. Its pulsations are palpable against the humerus between the axillary folds

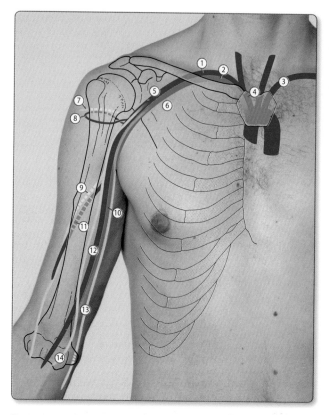

Figure 4.7 Main neurovasculature of the axilla and arm. ① Right subclavian artery, ② right subclavian vein, ③ left subclavian artery, ④ brachiocephalic trunk, ⑤ axillary artery and approximate position of brachial plexus, ⑥ axillary vein, ⑦ axillary nerve, ⑧ circumflex humeral arteries, ⑨ radial nerve, ⑩ brachial vein, ⑪ profunda brachii artery, ⑫ brachial artery, ⑬ ulnar nerve, ⑭ median nerve.

- The **circumflex humeral arteries** branch from the axillary artery ~ 5 cm inferior to the acromion and pass around the humeral surgical neck. The vessels and axillary nerve should be identified and avoided during a lateral surgical approach to the shoulder

- The **brachial artery** is a continuation of the axillary artery at the lower border of teres major (posterior axillary fold). It passes inferiorly in the groove between biceps and triceps and sits close to the medial humerus where its pulsations can be felt. Distally it sits anterior to the medial humeral supracondylar ridge and epicondyle
- The **profunda brachii artery** branches off the brachial just below latissimus dorsi (posterior axillary fold) and curves around the humeral spiral groove with the radial nerve

Veins

Deep veins The subclavian and axillary veins follow similar courses to their respective arteries (**Figure 4.7**). The subclavian vein sits anterior to the artery. The axillary vein is located anteroinferior to the artery proximally, and anteromedial to it distally. The subclavian artery is therefore at risk of perforation during subclavian vein cannulation.

Superficial veins The main superficial veins of the arm are the cephalic and basilic (**Figure 4.8**). Both are accompanied in the distal arm by medial or lateral cutaneous nerves of the forearm, which can be damaged during cannulation or phlebotomy.
- The **cephalic vein** passes proximally along the groove lateral to biceps, then through the deltopectoral groove to the infraclavicular fossa
- The **basilic vein** passes proximally along the groove medial to biceps. It travels deep around mid-arm level and at the lower border of the posterior axillary fold, it joins the brachial vein to form the axillary vein

4.2 Elbow, cubital fossa and forearm

Bones, joints and ligaments

Knowledge of the normal features and alignment of bones at the elbow helps with identification of joint lines, injection sites, nerve positions and diagnosis of dislocation/fracture (**Figures 4.9** and **4.10**).

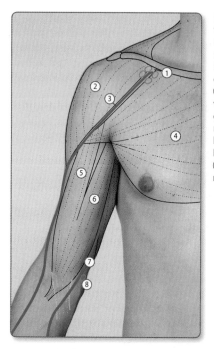

Figure 4.8 Superficial veins and lymph nodes of the arm and shoulder region. (1) Infraclavicular fossa/ deltopectoral triangle, (2) deltoid, (3) cephalic vein in deltopectoral groove, (4) pectoralis major, (5) biceps long head, (6) biceps short head, (7) basilic vein, (8) cubital lymph nodes.

Humerus

Three features of the distal humeral shaft are easily palpable.

- The **medial epicondyle** is the bony prominence on the medial elbow. Regional pain/tenderness can indicate pathology of the common flexor tendon (Golfer's elbow). The ulnar nerve sits posteriorly and can be injured by fracture
- The **lateral epicondyle** is the bony prominence on the posterolateral elbow, sat posterior to the forearm extensor muscle mass. Regional pain/tenderness can indicate pathology of the common extensor tendon (Tennis elbow)
- The **capitulum** sits medial to the lateral epicondyle and articulates inferiorly with the radial head

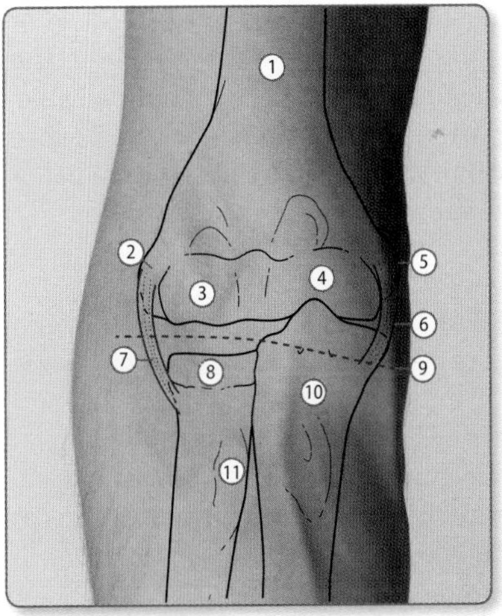

Figure 4.9 Elbow joint: anterior view. (1) Humeral shaft, (2) lateral epicondyle, (3) capitulum, (4) trochlea, (5) medial epicondyle, (6) medial collateral ligament, (7) lateral collateral ligament, (8) radial head, (9) elbow joint line, (10) ulna, (11) radial tuberosity.

Ulna

The **olecranon** process of the ulna is the raised prominence of bone located on the posterior elbow between the humeral epicondyles. The olecranon can be avulsed by triceps following a fall onto an outstretched limb, and displaced olecranon fractures can damage the medially located ulnar nerve. The posterior border of the ulna is palpable in its entirety from the olecranon to the ulna head at the medial wrist.

Regional alignment The apex of the olecranon normally aligns with the humeral epicondyles in full elbow extension and forms an equilateral triangle with the humeral epicondyles in 90° elbow flexion. Alterations of this alignment can indicate fracture or dislocation.

Radius

The radial head occupies the indented region on the posterior aspect of the elbow between the olecranon and

> ### Clinical insight
>
> The olecranon is covered by a subcutaneous bursa, which can become painfully inflamed and severely swollen in olecranon bursitis.

the forearm extensor muscle group. Fractures of the head or neck can damage the nearby posterior interosseous nerve. The proximal radial shaft is covered in muscle and is not palpable. Distally the lateral and posterior sides of the shaft are palpable. The horizontal groove of the radiohumeral joint can be palpated proximal to the radial head.

Joints

Elbow The elbow joint is the articulation of the humerus with the ulna and radius (**Figure 4.10**). The horizontal radiohumeral joint line is located ~ 2 cm inferior to the lateral epicondyle and is felt as an indentation between the radial head and humeral capitulum. The ulnerohumeral joint line slopes inferomedially and passes from the radiohumeral joint line to a point ~ 2.5 cm below the medial epicondyle.

The anconeus triangle marks the region used for elbow joint aspiration/injection. The triangle is a bounded by the lateral humeral epicondyle, the ulna olecranon and the radial head, and is covered by the anconeus muscle.

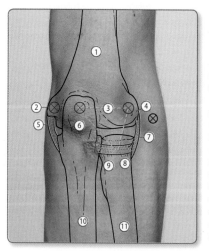

Figure 4.10 Elbow joint: posterior view. ① Humeral shaft, ② medial epicondyle, ③ borders of anconeus triangle (blue), ④ lateral epicondyle, ⑤ medial collateral ligament, ⑥ olecranon, ⑦ lateral collateral ligament, ⑧ annular ligament surrounding radial head, ⑨ radial neck, ⑩ posterior border of ulna, ⑪ radial shaft, Ⓧ horizontal alignment of the epicondyles and olecranon during elbow extension, Ⓧ forearm extensor muscle mass.

Superior radioulnar joint The proximal articulation between the radial head and ulna is palpable medial to the radial head. The radial head is kept in place by the annular ligament. Excess traction on a child's upper limb can subluxate the joint leading to a loss of normal alignment (Nursemaid's elbow).

Ligaments

The elbow and radioulnar joints are supported by strong ligaments that are palpable between their attachment points.

- The **lateral/radial collateral ligament** connects the lateral epicondyle to the radial annular ligament
- The **medial/ulnar collateral ligament** is broad and connects the medial epicondyle to the proximal ulna

Muscles, tendons and regions

The muscles and tendons of the forearm act on the elbow, wrist and digits and serve as good markers of underlying neurovascular structures.

Extensor muscles

A group of superficial extensor muscles share a common tendinous origin from the lateral epicondyle (**Figure 4.11, Table 4.3**). Pain/tenderness over the region indicates tendinitis/tennis elbow.

Muscle	Surface marking/route
Extensor carpi ulnaris	Passes distally toward the medial side of the ulnar head and styloid process
Extensor digiti minimi	Passes distally over the posterior of the ulna head towards digit 5
Extensor digitorum	Passes down the centre of the posterior forearm toward the midpoint of the wrist
Extensor carpi radialis brevis	Passes distally to the lateral side of the dorsal radial tubercle, toward the base of metacarpal 3

Table 4.3 Common extensor tendon muscles of the forearm.

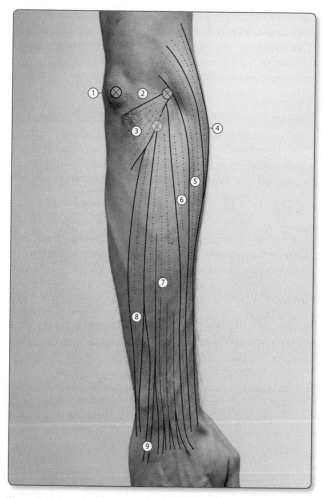

Figure 4.11 Superficial extensor muscles of the posterior forearm.
(1) Medial epicondyle, (2) borders of anconeus triangle (blue), (3) anconeus,
(4) brachioradialis, (5) extensor carpi radialis longus, (6) extensor carpi radialis
brevis, (7) extensor digitorum and extensor indicis, (8) extensor carpi ulnaris,
(9) extensor digiti minimi, (X) olecranon, (X) lateral epicondyle, (X) radial head.

Extensor pollicis brevis and abductor pollicis longus These pass inferolaterally from the middle of the posterior forearm toward the base of metacarpal 1. Both tendons can be felt passing over the tendons of extensor carpi radialis longus and brevis ~ 5 cm proximal to the radial styloid process (**Figure 4.22**)

Anconeus This passes over the posterior elbow from the lateral epicondyle to the lateral olecranon. It covers the anconeus triangle, the needle insertion site for the elbow

Extensor carpi radialis longus This travels alongside extensor carpi radialis brevis, passing distally from just above the lateral epicondyle toward the base of metacarpal 2.

Flexor muscles

A group of superficial flexor muscles share a common tendinous origin from the medial humeral epicondyle (**Figure 4.12**). Regional pain or tenderness, especially to palpation, indicates tendinitis/Golfer's elbow, which can be treated via an epicondylar injection of steroid. The group includes (**Table 4.4**):

Flexor digitorum profundus This passes inferiorly from the radius to the middle of the wrist under the cover of flexor digitorum superficialis.

Brachioradialis This passes down the anterolateral forearm, from the lateral supracondylar ridge to the lateral side of the distal radius. It is best seen in midpronation and resisted elbow flexion. Tapping the tendon tests a C5 and C6 reflex (radial nerve).

Cubital fossa

The cubital fossa is a triangular-shaped region located anterior to the elbow (**Figure 4.12**). The fossa is bordered:
- Laterally by brachioradialis
- Medially by pronator teres
- Superiorly by a line between the humeral epicondyles

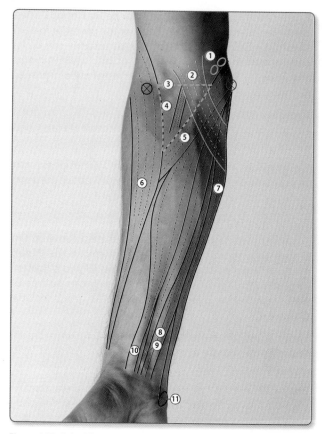

Figure 4.12 Cubital fossa and superficial flexor muscles of the anterior forearm. ① Cubital lymph nodes, ② bicipital aponeurosis, ③ borders of cubital fossa (blue), ④ biceps tendon, ⑤ pronator teres, ⑥ brachioradialis, ⑦ flexor carpi ulnaris, ⑧ flexor digitorum superficialis, ⑨ palmaris longus, ⑩ flexor carpi radialis, ⑪ pisiform, Ⓧ lateral epicondyle, Ⓧ medial epicondyle.

• Anteriorly (roof) by skin, deep fascia and biceps aponeurosis
The cubital fossa contains or is related to the structures listed in **Table 4.5** and shown in **Figure 4.13**:

Muscle	Surface marking/route
Pronator teres	Passes inferolaterally to the midpoint of the radius. Best palpated with the forearm in resisted pronation
Flexor carpi radialis	Passes inferolaterally towards the base of the thumb/thenar palmar crease. Its prominent tendon is seen on the lateral wrist. The radial artery sits immediately lateral to the tendon
Flexor carpi ulnaris	Passes inferiorly towards pisiform. The ulnar artery and nerve are located deep to the muscle proximally and lateral to it distally
Flexor digitorum superficialis	Passes toward the middle of the wrist, deep to palmaris longus and flexor carpi radialis. The tendons are palpable during finger flexion/extension
Palmaris longus	Thin muscle overlying flexor digitorum superficialis. Distally it landmarks the median nerve, which sits deep or lateral to it

Table 4.4 Common flexor tendon muscles of the forearm.

Structure	Surface marking/route
Biceps tendon	Passes distally through the central fossa. Tapping the tendon tests a C5 and C6 reflex
Brachial artery	Posteromedial to the biceps tendon. Its pulsation is felt deep to the bicipital aponeurosis, where it is auscultated during blood-pressure measurement and is at risk during venous cannulation
Median nerve	Medial to the brachial artery. Can be blocked medial to the arterial pulsation and 1–2 cm proximal to the elbow skin crease
Radial nerve	Sits in the groove between biceps tendon and brachio-radialis, ~ 1 cm lateral to biceps tendon. Can be blocked in the groove ~ 1–2 cm proximal to the elbow skin crease
Bicipital aponeurosis	Fibrous band passing inferomedially from biceps across the fossa roof. Medially it forms a sharp ridge. Protects the brachial artery and median nerve during venous cannulation
Cubital lymph nodes	Sit close to the basilic vein and medial epicondyle. Receive lymph from the hand and forearm. Enlarge during infection, e.g. cellulitis
Cephalic vein	Passes proximally over the lateral fossa
Basilic vein	Passes proximally over the medial fossa

Table 4.5 Contents and relations of the cubital fossa.

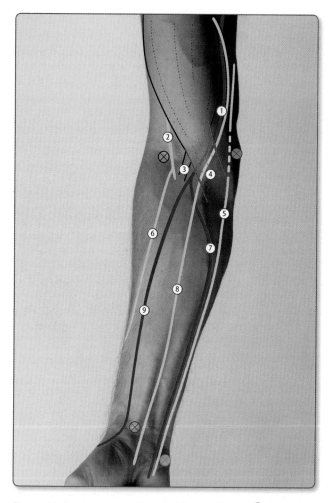

Figure 4.13 Neurovasculature of the cubital fossa and forearm. ① Brachial artery, ② radial nerve, ③ biceps tendon, ④ biceps aponeurosis, ⑤ ulnar nerve, ⑥ superficial branch of radial nerve, ⑦ ulnar artery, ⑧ median nerve, ⑨ radial artery, Ⓧ lateral epicondyle, Ⓧ medial epicondyle, Ⓧ flexor carpi radialis tendon, Ⓧ pisiform and flexor carpi ulnaris tendon.

Neurovasculature
Arteries

The brachial artery passes into the cubital fossa deep to the biceps aponeurosis and medial to its tendon (**Figures 4.13** and **4.14**). It bifurcates into the ulnar and radial arteries at the level of the radial head (~ 2 cm distal to a line passing through the humeral epicondyles).

- The **ulnar artery** passes inferomedially to meet the ulnar nerve deep to flexor carpi ulnaris about one third of the way down the forearm. Both then pass inferiorly toward the lateral side of the pisiform along the line of the ulna. The ulnar artery can sometimes be palpated at the wrist, lateral to pisiform and the tendon of flexor carpi ulnaris
- The **radial artery** passes inferolaterally to the wrist along a line joining the biceps tendon to a point midway between the tendon of flexor carpi radialis and the radial styloid process where it is easily palpated and accessed (blood gas/angiography/dialysis). Throughout most of the forearm it sits deep to brachioradialis

Nerves

Median nerve This nerve travels down the forearm along a line passing from the medial side of the brachial artery in the cubital fossa to

> ### Clinical insight
>
> Allen test for patency of hand blood supply occludes the radial and ulnar arteries at the wrist. Each is released individually whilst monitoring hand reperfusion.

the middle of the wrist, deep or just lateral to the tendon of palmaris longus. It sits deep to flexor digitorum superficialis. Penetrating wrist injury can damage the nerve and knowledge of its position guides the choice of surgical incision site during carpal tunnel decompression.

Ulnar nerve This nerve travels down the anterior forearm along a line joining the medial epicondyle with the lateral side of the pisiform bone. Proximally it sits deep to flexor carpi ulnaris and distally it sits lateral to it.

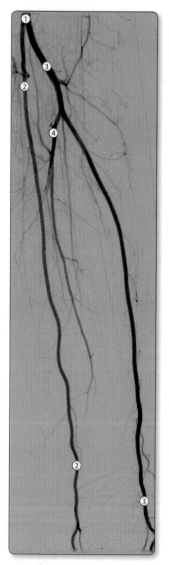

Figure 4.14 Arteriogram of the right forearm. (1) Brachial artery, (2) radial artery, (3) ulnar artery, (4) common interosseous artery.

Radial nerve This nerve is situated in the groove between the biceps tendon and brachioradialis, ~ 1 cm lateral to biceps tendon. Here it can be anaesthetised or injured during arthroscopic elbow procedures. It passes close to the radiohumeral joint and divides into superficial and deep branches:

- The **deep (posterior interosseous) branch** winds around the lateral radial shaft ~ 2–3 cm distal to the radial head, where it can be injured in radial fracture, radioulnar joint dislocation or surgical incision. It descends the posterior forearm along a line passing from the radial head toward extensor compartment 4 of the wrist
- The **superficial branch** passes distally deep to brachioradialis and then becomes superficial on the dorsolateral forearm ~ 5–8 cm proximal to the radial styloid. The nerve can be blocked at this location anaesthetising skin over the first dorsal interosseous and dorsum of digits 1–3

Superficial veins and cutaneous nerves

The superficial veins of the upper limb originate from the dorsal venous network of the hand, where access is simple (**Figures 4.15** and **4.16**). Note, several cutaneous nerves run close to the superficial veins and can therefore be damaged during cannulation (**Table 4.6**). Regional cutaneous nerves are also at risk during medial or lateral surgical approaches to the elbow.

4.3 Wrist and hand

Bones, joints and ligaments

Ulna and radius

Radial styloid process This projects distally from the lateral side of the distal radius (**Figure 4.17**). It is palpable proximally in the anatomical snuffbox. The dorsal radial (Lister's) tubercle is a bony prominence located on the dorsal radius in line with the web space between digits 2 and 3. It helps landmark the extensor tendon compartments of the wrist and is a landmark for wrist injection. Falling onto an outstretched hand can fracture and displace the distal radius dorsally (Colles' fracture/ dinner fork deformity), whereas falling onto the dorsum of a flexed wrist can displace the radius anteriorly (Smith's fracture).

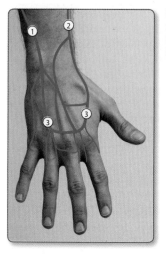

Figure 4.15 Dorsal venous network of the hand. ① Basilic vein, ② cephalic vein, ③ dorsal venous network (arch).

Vein	Origin	Surface marking and nerve association
Cephalic	Lateral side of dorsal venous network of the hand	Passes over the anatomical snuffbox alongside the superficial radial nerve. Ascends the dorsolateral forearm distally then moves anteriorly to pass over the lateral cubital fossa alongside the lateral cutaneous nerve of the forearm
Basilic	Medial side of dorsal venous network of the hand	Ascends the dorsomedial surface of the distal forearm. Moves anteriorly to pass over the medial cubital fossa alongside the medial cutaneous nerve of the forearm, or its anterior and posterior branches
Median cubital	Cephalic vein ~ 5 cm distal to the lateral epicondyle	Passes superomedially over the cubital fossa and joins the basilic vein around medial epicondyle level. Commonly used for cannulation/phlebotomy
Median of forearm	Palmar veins on anterior forearm	Ascends the centre of the anterior forearm to join the median cubital or basilic vein proximally. Can run alongside the lateral cutaneous nerve of the forearm

Table 4.6 Superficial veins and cutaneous nerves of the upper limb.

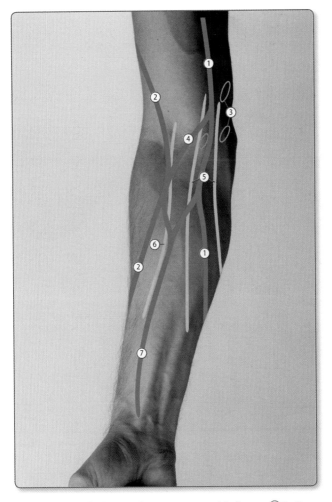

Figure 4.16 Superficial veins and cutaneous nerves of the forearm. ① Basilic vein, ② cephalic vein, ③ cubital lymph nodes, ④ median cubital vein, ⑤ medial cutaneous nerve of the forearm (anterior and posterior branches), ⑥ lateral cutaneous nerve of the forearm, ⑦ median vein of the forearm.

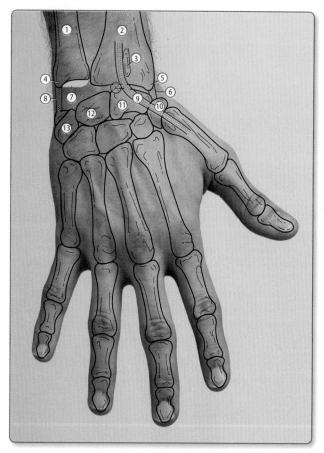

Figure 4.17 Osteology and ligaments of the posterior wrist and hand.
① Ulna, ② radius, ③ dorsal radial (Lister's) tubercle, ④ ulna styloid process, ⑤ radial styloid process, ⑥ radial collateral ligament, ⑦ articular disc (triangular fibrocartilage), ⑧ ulna collateral ligament, ⑨ tendon of extensor pollicis longus, ⑩ trapezium, ⑪ scaphoid, ⑫ lunate, ⑬ triquetrum, ⊗ wrist injection/aspiration site.

Ulnar head This is rounded and easily palpated on the dorsomedial wrist. The ulna styloid process projects distally from the medial side of the head. Note, the tip of the radial styloid is normally located ~ 1 cm distal to the tip of the ulna styloid. Variation in this arrangement can indicate a proximal fracture or dislocation.

Wrist joint

The wrist joint line is marked by the proximal wrist crease. It can be palpated immediately distal to both the ulna and radial styloid processes. The joint can be injected/aspirated via the indented space located just distal and medial to the dorsal radial tubercle and medial to the extensor pollicis longus tendon.

Ligaments and triangular fibrocartilage complex Two of the ligaments supporting the wrist are palpable medially and laterally between their attachment points. Pain on palpation indicates injury and both can be injected if required.
- The **radial collateral ligament** passes from the radial styloid process to the scaphoid along anatomical snuffbox floor
- The **ulnar collateral ligament** passes from the ulna styloid process to the triquetrum. The triangular fibrocartilage complex (articular disc) of the wrist sits deep to the ligament and can be tender/painful to palpation when injured

Carpal bones

The carpal bones are located in the proximal hand (**Figures 4.17–4.19**). Several can be identified and act as landmarks for neurovascular structures and the flexor retinaculum forming the carpal tunnel's roof. Note, carpal bones can be fractured by a fall onto an outstretched hand (**Table 4.7**).

Metacarpals, phalanges and joints

Metacarpals These are palpable on the dorsal hand (**Figures 4.18** and **4.19**). Their bases articulate with the carpal bones at the carpometacarpal joints, along a line ~ 2–3 cm distal to the dorsal radial tubercle. The first carpometacarpal joint is palpable in the distal anatomical snuffbox. It can become painful from overuse or osteoarthritis. To enable injection of the first carpometacarpal joint space it is opened out via thumb flexion and distraction (pulling).

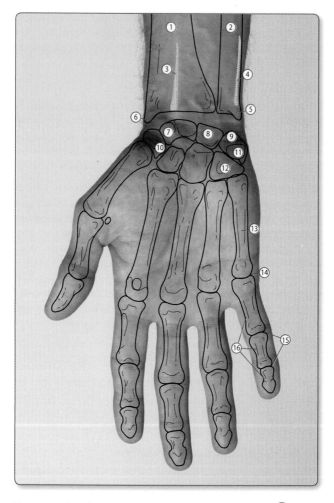

Figure 4.18 Osteology and ligaments of the anterior wrist and hand. ① Radius, ② ulna, ③ line of flexor carpi radialis tendon, ④ line of flexor carpi ulnaris tendon, ⑤ ulna styloid process, ⑥ radial styloid process, ⑦ scaphoid tubercle, ⑧ lunate, ⑨ triquetrum, ⑩ trapezium tubercle, ⑪ pisiform, ⑫ hook of hamate, ⑬ metacarpal bones, ⑭ metacarpophalangeal joint, ⑮ interphalangeal joints (proximal and distal), ⑯ phalangeal bones (proximal, middle and distal).

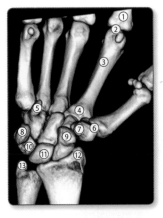

Figure 4.19 3D rendered CT image of the bones of the anterior wrist and hand (carpal tunnel). ① Proximal phalanx, ② 2nd metacarpophalangeal joint, ③ 2nd metacarpal, ④ base of 2nd metacarpal, ⑤ hook of hamate, ⑥ 1st carpometacarpal joint, ⑦ trapezium tubercle, ⑧ pisiform, ⑨ scaphoid tubercle, ⑩ triquetrum (floor of carpal tunnel), ⑪ lunate (floor of carpal tunnel), ⑫ radial styloid process, ⑬ ulnar styloid process.

Bone/feature	Surface marking	Relevance
Scaphoid	Floor of the anatomical snuffbox immediately distal to the radial styloid	Tenderness to palpation/wrist dorsiflexion can indicate fracture
Scaphoid tubercle	Palm of the hand where flexor carpi radialis meets the thenar muscles	Median nerve sits medially. Flexor retinaculum attachment point
Trapezium tubercle	Palm of the hand, immediately distal to the scaphoid tubercle	Flexor retinaculum attachment point
Pisiform	Rounded bone of the anteromedial wrist. Sits in line with the distal wrist crease and flexor carpi ulnaris tendon	Ulnar artery and nerve sit laterally. Flexor retinaculum attachment point
Hook of hamate	Palpable in the palm both 2 cm distal and 2 cm lateral to pisiform	Ulnar artery and nerve sit medially. Flexor retinaculum attachment point
Triquetrum	Palpable on the medial surface of the wrist just distal to the ulna styloid	Commonly fractured carpal bone

Table 4.7 Carpal bones of the hand.

Metacarpophalangeal joint line This is palpable on the dorsal hand, either side of the extensor tendon. The rounded metacarpal heads are palpable at the knuckle during digit flexion. The joints can be injected if painful or inflamed via a medial or lateral approach.

> ### Clinical insight
>
> With the fist clenched the middle phalanx of digits 2–4 point toward the scaphoid. Deviation from this alignment indicates a rotational displacement of a digit.

Phalanges These are palpable on the dorsal hand. The base of each phalanx forms the widest part of the interphalangeal joint. Each joint line is palpable proximal to the widest part on the medial and lateral sides of the fingers. The interphalangeal joints can be injected via a lateral or medial approach.

Muscles, tendons and regions

Anatomical snuffbox

The anatomical snuffbox is an indented region located lateral to the wrist (**Figures 4.20** and **4.21**). It is best seen with the wrist and thumb extended. The snuffbox is bounded:

- Anteriorly by the tendons of abductor pollicis longus and extensor pollicis brevis
- Posteriorly by the tendon of extensor pollicis longus

The floor of the snuffbox is formed by palpable bones, which, from proximal to distal, are:

- Radial styloid process
- Scaphoid, in the deepest part of the fossa
- Trapezium and the 1st carpometacarpal joint
- Base of metacarpal 1

Contents

- The **radial artery** passes posteriorly over the distal snuffbox floor deep to all tendons then passes through the proximal part of the 1st dorsal interosseous to enter the palm. Care needs to be taken to avoid the artery during 1st carpometacarpal joint injection

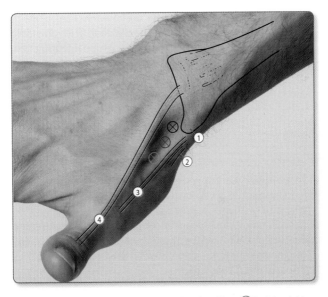

Figure 4.20 Borders and bones of the anatomical snuffbox. ① Radial styloid process, ② abductor pollicis longus tendon, ③ extensor pollicis brevis tendon, ④ extensor pollicis longus tendon, ⊗ scaphoid, ⊗ trapezium, ⊗ base of 1st metacarpal.

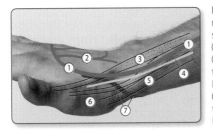

Figure 4.21 Neurovascular relations of the anatomical snuffbox. ① Cephalic vein, ② dorsal venous network, ③ extensor pollicis longus tendon, ④ superficial branch of radial nerve, ⑤ abductor pollicis longus tendon, ⑥ extensor pollicis brevis, ⑦ radial artery.

- The **cephalic vein** passes proximally over the centre of the snuffbox. The vein is often used for cannulation and is referred to as houseman's (or intern's) vein as its position is relatively consistent

- The **superficial branch of the radial nerve** runs close to the cephalic vein and onto the dorsal hand. It is vulnerable during regional cannulation. Injury causes pain, numbness or paraesthesia in the skin covering the first dorsal interosseous and the dorsal surfaces of the lateral 3.5 digits.

> ## Clinical insight
>
> Smooth, round, firm and non-tender swellings known as ganglia can develop on tendons of the wrist/hand. They commonly occur on the extensor carpi radialis brevis tendon.

Extensor compartments of the wrist

The extensor tendons pass over the wrist in six compartments (**Figure 4.22**). Knowledge of the compartments and their contents helps in wrist pain diagnosis. For example, de Quervain tenosynovitis causes compartment 1 pain, over the radial styloid, and can be treated via steroid injection. The injection site sits in the gap between the two tendons of the compartment (**Table 4.8**).

Dorsal hand

Digital extensor tendons These can be traced from extensor compartments 4 and 5 to the proximal phalanges of the digits after which they spread out to form the flattened extensor expansion.

Dorsal interossei These are longitudinal masses of muscle located between adjacent metacarpals. Thumb adduction makes the first dorsal interosseous prominent. Interosseus wasting occurs after ulnar/T1 nerve injury resulting in weak digit abduction and adduction and guttering/indentations between the metacarpals.

Palmar (volar) wrist and hand

Palmaris longus This is a superficial relatively thin midline muscle that is best seen with the tips of the digits and thumb opposed and the wrist in slight flexion (**Figure 4.23**). It can be absent. The median nerve is located immediately deep, or just lateral, to the tendon therefore surgical approaches to the tunnel are made medial to the tendon.

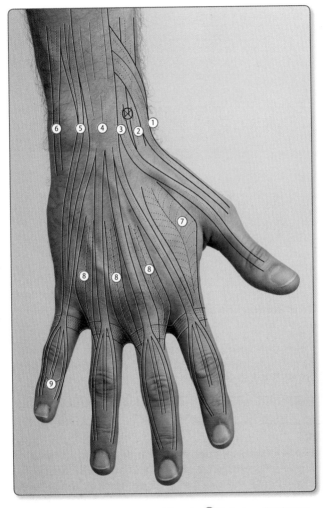

Figure 4.22 Extensor compartments of the wrist. (1) Abductor pollicis longus and extensor pollicis brevis (compartment 1), (2) extensor carpi radialis longus and brevis (compartment 2), (3) extensor pollicis longus (compartment 3), (4) extensor digitorum and indicis (compartment 4), (5) extensor digiti minimi (compartment 5), (6) extensor carpi ulnaris (compartment 6), (7) 1st dorsal interosseous muscle, (8) dorsal interosseous muscles, (9) extensor expansion of digit, (X) dorsal radial tubercle.

Compartment	Surface marking and content
1	Lateral to the radial styloid process. Contains abductor pollicis longus and extensor pollicis brevis. Subject to a painful tenosynovitis the cause of which is idiopathic (de Quervain) or overuse (mobile phone thumb)
2	Immediately lateral to the dorsal radial tubercle. Contains extensor carpi radialis longus and brevis passing distally to the bases of metacarpals 2 and 3
3	Immediately medial to the dorsal radial tubercle. Contains extensor pollicis longus, which can wear on the radial tubercle and rupture
4	Situated between compartment 3 and the ulna head. Contains extensor digitorum and indicis passing to the digits
5	On the posterior aspect of the ulna head. Contains extensor digiti minimi
6	On the medial surface of the ulna head and styloid process. Contains extensor carpi ulnaris, which can wear on the styloid process and rupture

Table 4.8 Extensor compartments of the dorsal wrist.

Flexor carpi ulnaris This passes over medial wrist and attaches to the pisiform bone, where its tendon can be seen and palpated. The ulnar artery and nerve sit laterally.

Flexor carpi radialis This forms the most lateral tendon of the anterior wrist, which passes towards the base of the thenar palmar crease. The radial artery is located laterally.

Flexor digitorum superficialis and profundus These sit between flexor carpi radialis and ulnaris and pass through the carpal tunnel and palm to the digits. Flexor digitorum superficialis attaches to the sides of the middle phalanx and flexor digitorum profundus attaches to the base of the distal phalanx.

The thenar and hypothenar eminences These are prominent masses of muscle located on the lateral and medial palm, respectively. Both eminences contain three muscles, an abductor

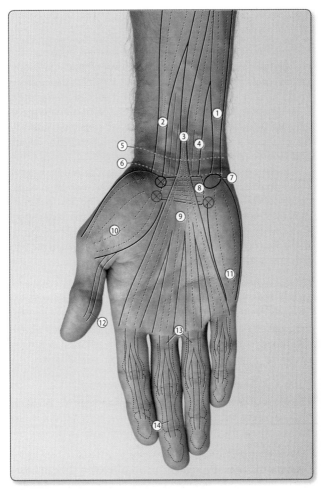

Figure 4.23 Muscles and bony landmarks of the anterior wrist and hand.
① Flexor carpi ulnaris, ② flexor carpi radialis, ③ palmaris longus, ④ flexor digitorum superficialis, ⑤ proximal wrist crease, ⑥ distal wrist crease, ⑦ pisiform, ⑧ flexor retinaculum/transverse carpal ligament (roof of carpal tunnel), ⑨ palmar aponeurosis, ⑩ thenar eminence, ⑪ hypothenar eminence, ⑫ tendon of flexor pollicis longus, ⑬ tendons of flexor digitorum superficialis, ⑭ tendons of flexor digitorum profundus, Ⓧ scaphoid tubercle, Ⓧ trapezium tubercle, Ⓧ hook of hamate.

and a flexor overlying an opposer muscle, that act on the thumb (thenar) or 5th digit (hypothenar).

Carpal tunnel The carpal tunnel is formed between the U-shape of the carpal bones and the flexor retinaculum/transverse carpal ligament (**Figure 4.19** and **4.23**). Its entrance aligns with the distal wrist crease and its roof, the flexor retinaculum, is landmarked between pisiform and hook of hamate medially, and the tubercles of the scaphoid and trapezium laterally. It contains the digital flexor tendons, common flexor sheath and median nerve.

Carpal tunnel syndrome compresses the median nerve resulting in pain in the lateral digits, which is worse at night, and thenar muscle wasting/weakness rendering dextrous tasks difficult. The tunnel can be injected with anaesthetic or steroid via a site located medial to palmaris longus and 1 cm proximal to the distal wrist crease. The needle is directed toward the ring finger at a 30° angle to the skin and advanced 2 cm.

Palmar aponeurosis The fibrous aponeurosis covers the palm and protects it from penetrating injury. It begins at the flexor retinaculum and fans out to blend with the fibrous sheaths of the digits. Dupuytren contracture is an idiopathic thickened and shortening of the aponeurosis that causes a flexion deformity of the hand and metacarpals. It can become debilitating.

Synovial sheaths and spaces of the hand
The synovial sheaths and spaces of the hand can act as routes for infection spread and associated swelling (**Figure 4.24**). Knowledge of their location and communication is therefore important.

Synovial sheaths Elongated synovial sheaths (bursa) cover the flexor tendons. The bursa begin 1–2 cm proximal to the proximal flexor wrist crease and pass through the carpal tunnel into the palm.
- The **ulna bursa** covers the flexor tendons of digits 2–5 in to the proximal palm. The bursa covering the tendon to digit 5 extends to its distal phalanx

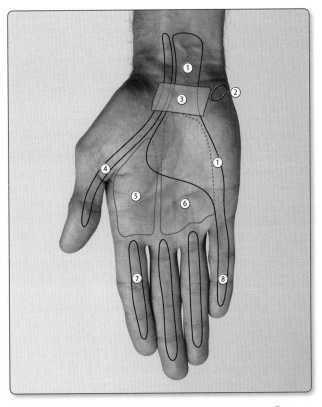

Figure 4.24 Synovial bursae/sheaths and spaces of the palmar hand. (1) Ulna bursa, (2) pisiform, (3) flexor retinaculum/transverse carpal ligament (roof of carpal tunnel), (4) radial bursa, (5) thenar space, (6) midpalmar space, (7) digital synovial sheaths, (8) digital synovial sheath of digit 5 communicating with ulna bursa.

- The **radial bursa** covers the flexor pollicis longus tendon and follows it to the distal phalanx of digit 1 (thumb)
- The **digital synovial sheaths** cover the digital flexor tendons as they pass distally over the phalanges of digits 2–4

Palmar spaces The midpalmar and thenar spaces are located deep in the palm and are separated by a fibrous septum that joins the palmar aponeurosis to the 3rd metacarpal.

- The **midpalmar space** sits deep to the flexor tendons of digits 3–5, and extends from the carpal tunnel to the metacarpal heads. It can communicate with the anterior forearm via the carpal tunnel
- The **thenar space** sits between the 3rd metacarpal and the thenar eminence, deep to the flexor tendon of digit 2

Pulp spaces and nail fold The proximal and lateral nail folds flank the nail in a U-shape. The proximal fold meets the nail at the eponychium (**Figure 4.25**). The digital pulp spaces sit over the palmar surfaces of the phalanges and are separated by connective tissue (**Figure 4.26**). Infections of a pulp space (felon) or nail fold (paronychia) tend to remain localised.

Clinical insight

Trigger finger (stenosing tenosynovitis) causes passive digit flexion with a tender palpable nodule on the flexor tendon located near the proximal digital crease.

A wing block can be used to anaesthetise the nail bed. The needle is inserted 3 mm proximal to the point of intersection of the proximal and lateral nail folds. Anaesthetic is injected along the proximal skin fold then along the lateral fold and the procedure repeated on the opposite side.

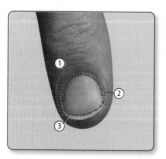

Figure 4.25 Nails folds and nail bed. ① Proximal nail fold, ② lateral nail fold, ③ border of nail bed.

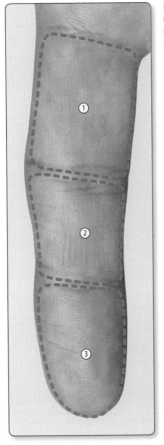

Figure 4.26 Digital pulp spaces.
① Proximal digital pulp space,
② middle digital pulp space,
③ distal digital pulp space.

Neurovasculature

Nerves

Median nerve This nerve passes through the carpal tunnel and into the palm along a plane aligned with the tendon of palmaris longus (**Figure 4.27**). It branches ~ 2–3 cm distal to the distal wrist crease.

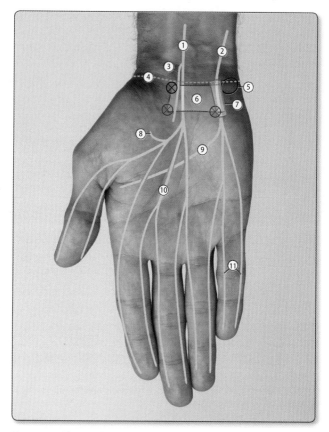

Figure 4.27 The carpal tunnel, Guyon's canal and nerves of the palmar (volar) hand. ① Median nerve, ② ulnar nerve, ③ palmar branch of median nerve, ④ distal wrist crease, ⑤ pisiform, ⑥ flexor retinaculum/transverse carpal ligament (roof of the carpal tunnel), ⑦ Guyon's canal, ⑧ recurrent branch of median nerve, ⑨ deep branch of ulnar nerve, ⑩ common palmar digital sensory nerves, ⑪ palmar digital sensory nerves, Ⓧ scaphoid tubercle, Ⓧ trapezium tubercle, Ⓧ hook of hamate.

- The **palmar digital branches** ascend the medial and lateral sides of digits 1–3 and the lateral side of digit 4

- The **recurrent branch** turns back on itself to enter and supply the thenar muscles

The palmar cutaneous branch travels superficial to the flexor retinaculum just lateral to the plane of palmaris longus

Ulnar nerve This nerve passes into the palm lateral to pisiform and medial to the hook of hamate through Guyon's canal. It gives off two branches ~ 1 cm distal to pisiform:

- The **superficial branch** sends palmar digital nerves along the sides of the medial 1.5 digits
- The **deep branch** curves laterally across the midpalmar space toward the thumb web space to innervate hand muscles

Guyon's canal This extends ~ 4 cm distal from the distal wrist crease between pisiform, hamate and the flexor retinaculum. It contains the ulnar nerve and artery. Both can be compressed by ganglia, fractures or abnormal anatomy resulting in sensory changes/pain over the medial 1.5 digits, weakness/wasting of the intrinsic hand muscles (except the thenar eminence) and clawing of digits 4 and 5.

Arteries

Ulnar artery This artery passes into the palm through Guyon's canal, lateral to the ulnar nerve and branches close to the hamate (**Figures 4.28** and **4.29**).

- The **deep branch** passes into the midpalmar space to join the deep palmar arch
- The **superficial palmar arch** curves laterally under the palmar aponeurosis and sends digital branches to the medial and lateral palmar sides of most digits. The arch extends distally to a horizontal plane drawn level with the distal surface of an extended thumb (**Figure 4.28**).

Radial artery The superficial palmar branch of the radial passes into the palm over the thenar muscles on a plane ~ 1 cm lateral to flexor carpi radialis to anastomose with the superficial palmar arch. The radial artery passes into the palm through the proximal part of the first dorsal interosseous and forms the deep palmar arch. The deep arch passes through both palmar spaces, on a plane ~ 2–3 cm proximal to the superficial palmar arch.

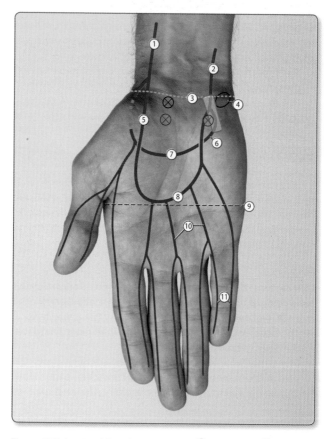

Figure 4.28 Arteries of the palmar (volar) hand. ① Radial artery, ② ulnar artery, ③ distal wrist crease, ④ pisiform, ⑤ superficial palmar branch of radial artery, ⑥ deep branch of ulnar artery, ⑦ deep palmar arch, ⑧ superficial palmar arch, ⑨ plane of extended thumb (distal extent of superficial arch), ⑩ common palmar digital arteries, ⑪ palmar digital arteries, Ⓧ scaphoid tubercle, Ⓧ trapezium tubercle, Ⓧ hook of hamate.

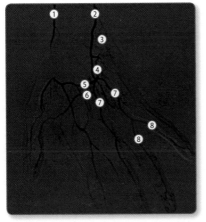

Figure 4.29 Arteriogram of the right hand. (1) Ulnar artery, (2) radial artery, (3) pisiform, (4) deep branch of ulnar artery, (5) deep palmar arch, (6) superficial palmar arch, (7) common palmar digital arteries, (8) palmar digital arteries.

Digital arteries and nerves These pass along the medial and lateral sides of both the palmar and dorsal surfaces of the digits toward the distal phalanx. Knowledge of this arrangement enables efficient digital block and avoidance of the arteries during invasive procedures. To carry out a digital block the needle is inserted perpendicular to the digit via the dorsal surface of the web space, near to the metacarpal heads, and advanced toward the palm enabling both dorsal and palmar digital branches to be anaesthetised. Both sides of the digit must be anaesthetised.

Lower limb

The lower limb is formed by the gluteal region, thigh, leg and foot. It articulates proximally with the pelvic girdle via the hip joint. The pelvic girdle is formed by the left and right hip bones and the sacrum. It contributes to the lower part of the trunk and encloses the greater and lesser pelves. The girdle connects the lower limb with the axial skeleton and transmits weight and locomotive forces between them.

Fascia and compartments

Strong deep fascia surrounds the limb and joins with bone via intermuscular septa thus forming compartments (**Table 5.1** and **Figures 5.1–5.3**). Increases in intracompartmental pressure (compartment syndrome) due to bleeds or infection are characterised by limb pain and varying levels of pallor, pulselessness, paraesthesia and paralysis.

Iliotibial tract/band

The fascia lata between the iliac crest and Gerdy's tubercle on the anterior surface of the lateral tibial condyle is thickened to form the iliotibial tract or band (**Figure 5.2**). The tract can be seen and felt over the lateral thigh and knee especially when weight bearing in knee flexion. Excess rubbing of the tract

Region	Fascia	Compartments
Gluteal	Gluteal	Gluteal
Thigh	Fascia lata/deep thigh	Anterior, posterior and medial
Leg	Crural/deep leg	Anterior, posterior and lateral
Foot	Dorsal fascia	Dorsal
	Plantar fascia	Medial, lateral, central and interosseous

Table 5.1 Fascia and compartments of the lower limb.

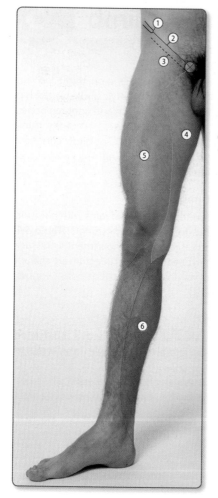

Figure 5.1 Lower limb compartments: antero-medial view. ① Anterior superior iliac spine, ② inguinal ligament, ③ anterior thigh (Holden's) skin crease, ④ medial thigh compartment, ⑤ anterior thigh compartment, ⑥ posterior leg compartment.

on the lateral femoral condyle can cause iliotibial tract/band syndrome, which is characterised by pain on movement and tenderness to palpation.

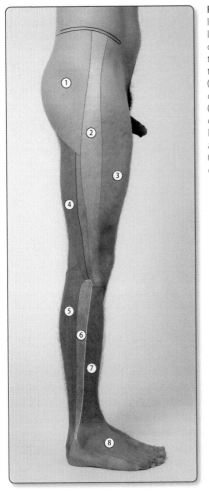

Figure 5.2 Lower limb compartments: lateral view. (1) Gluteal compartment, (2) iliotibial tract/band, (3) anterior thigh compartment, (4) posterior thigh compartment, (5) posterior leg compartment, (6) lateral leg compartment, (7) anterior leg compartment, (8) dorsal foot compartment.

Skin creases

Skin creases of the limb can be used to landmark compartments and joints.

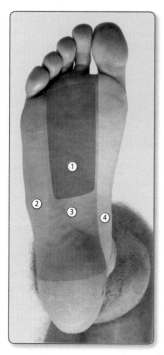

Figure 5.3 Compartments of the plantar foot. ① Interosseous foot compartment, ② lateral foot compartment, ③ central foot compartment, ④ medial foot compartment.

- The **anterior thigh (Holden's) crease** sits ~ 2–3 cm (two fingers breadth) distal to the inguinal ligament and is visible during hip flexion (**Figure 5.1**). It marks the junction between the fascia lata and Scarpa's abdominal fascia and therefore the inferior limit of infection/urine spread from the perineum/abdominal wall
- The **gluteal creases** pass almost horizontally across the lower gluteal region and mark the superior limit of the posterior thigh compartment (**Figure 5.4**)

5.1 Pelvic girdle, gluteal region and thigh

Bones, joints and ligaments

Pelvic girdle

Many of the features, joints and ligaments of the pelvic girdle are discussed in **Chapters 3, 6** and **7**. Several features such as the ischial tuberosity and anterior superior iliac spine are tendon attachment points and are therefore subject to avulsion fracture. Symptoms include sudden severe pain, bruising and swelling.

Greater and lesser sciatic foramen These are associated with major nerves and vessels. Piriformis sits posterior to the sacral plexus and divides the greater foramen into suprapiriform and infrapiriform parts. The foramen can be landmarked posteriorly via a line drawn between the posterior superior iliac spine and ischial tuberosity (**Table 5.2** and **Figures 5.4** and **5.5**).

Gluteal region injection Intramuscular gluteal region injection must avoid the major underlying neurovascular structures. Variability in regional size and shape necessitates the use of reliable bony landmarks. Two methods can be used (**Figure 5.5**). For both methods the injection is made into gluteus medius in the upper lateral part of the safe region.

- **Method 1:** the region is divided into quadrants using a vertical line through the highest point of the iliac crest and a horizontal line midway between the ischial tuberosity and the highest point of the iliac crest

Foramen	Surface markings	Communication and contents
Greater sciatic foramen (suprapiriform part)	One third of the way down the line joining the posterior superior iliac spine and ischial tuberosity	Pelvic cavity; superior gluteal neurovasculature; marks a needle insertion point for a sacral plexus block
Greater sciatic foramen (infrapiriform part)	Midpoint of the line joining the posterior superior iliac spine and ischial tuberosity	Pelvic cavity; inferior gluteal and pudendal neurovasculature; sciatic nerve; posterior cutaneous nerve of thigh
Lesser sciatic foramen	Two thirds of the way down the line joining the posterior superior iliac spine and ischial tuberosity	Ischioanal fossae; pudendal neurovasculature

Table 5.2 Surface markings, communications and content of the sciatic foramen.

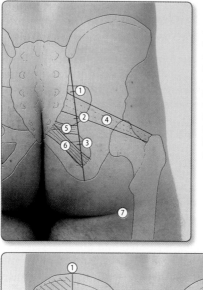

Figure 5.4 Osteology of the pelvic girdle and sciatic foramen. ① Suprapiriform part of greater sciatic foramen, ② infrapiriform part of greater sciatic foramen, ③ lesser sciatic foramen, ④ piriformis, ⑤ sacrospinous ligament, ⑥ sacrotuberous ligament, ⑦ gluteal crease.

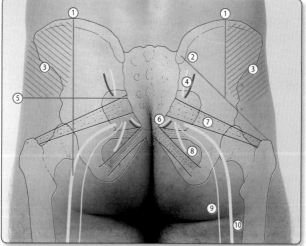

Figure 5.5 Gluteal region neurovasculature and injection sites. ① Vertical line through highest point of iliac crest, ② posterior superior iliac spine-greater trochanter line, ③ safe region for intramuscular injection, ④ superior gluteal nerve and artery, ⑤ horizontal plane midway between iliac crest and ischial tuberosity, ⑥ inferior gluteal nerve and artery, ⑦ piriformis, ⑧ pudendal nerve, ⑨ posterior cutaneous nerve of thigh, ⑩ sciatic nerve.

- **Method 2:** a vertical line passing through the highest point of the iliac crest is intersected with a line passing from the posterior superior iliac spine to the top of the greater trochanter

Femur

Several features of the femur can be palpated or landmarked (**Figure 5.6**):

- The **greater trochanter** can be palpated as a firm mass on the upper lateral thigh on a horizontal plane aligned with the pubic tubercle. Trochanteric bursitis can cause regional tenderness
- The **medial** and **lateral femoral condyles** can be palpated through the skin around the knee, especially during knee flexion. The epicondyles can be palpated above the condyles and deep palpation above the medial epicondyle reveals the prominent adductor tubercle
- The **shaft** sits deep to the thigh muscles. It passes inferomedially from a point ~ 2.5 cm medial to the greater trochanter to the midpoint of the patella. High impact forces are required to fracture a healthy femoral shaft

Patella

The patella articulates with the anterior of the femoral condyles and its margins and anterior surface are easily palpated. Its superiorly-located base attaches to the quadriceps tendon and its narrower inferiorly-located apex attaches to the patellar ligament and sits up to 2 cm above the knee joint line. Patella fractures cause anterior knee pain and swelling and are often displaced by quadriceps.

Hip joint

The hip joint is not palpable but can be landmarked via a point just below and lateral to the midpoint of the ingui-

> ### Clinical insight
>
> Femoral neck fractures result in the limb appearing shorter and externally rotated with pain and groin tenderness over the joint line.

nal ligament. Alternatively the joint centre sits ~ 2–4 cm vertically above the midpoint of a line joining the pubic tubercle to the upper part of the greater trochanter (**Figures 5.6** and **5.7**).

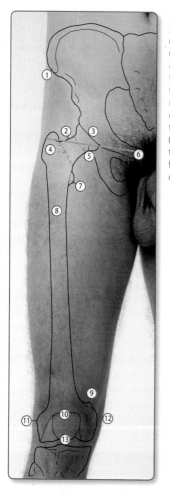

Figure 5.6 Osteology of the pelvic girdle, hip, femur and knee. ① Anterior superior iliac spine, ② femoral neck, ③ acetabulum overlying femoral head, ④ greater trochanter, ⑤ midpoint of pubic tubercle-greater trochanter line marking vertical plane of hip joint centre, ⑥ pubic tubercle-greater trochanter line, ⑦ lesser trochanter, ⑧ femoral shaft, ⑨ adductor tubercle, ⑩ base of patella, ⑪ lateral femoral condyle, ⑫ medial femoral condyle, ⑬ patellar apex.

In some subjects the joint sits on the midpoint of this line. Hip joint injection/aspiration can be carried out via a lateral approach using a site just above the greater trochanter or via an anterior approach using ultrasound.

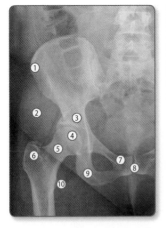

Figure 5.7 Radiograph of the right hip joint. ① Anterior superior iliac spine, ② gluteus medius and minimus, ③ margin of acetabulum, ④ femoral head, ⑤ femoral neck, ⑥ greater trochanter, ⑦ pubic tubercle, ⑧ pubic symphysis, ⑨ ischial tuberosity, ⑩ lesser trochanter.

Muscles, tendons and regions
Gluteal region
Gluteus maximus This is the largest and most superficial regional muscle (**Figure 5.8**). Its upper border passes inferolaterally from the iliac crest, ~ 5–7 cm superolateral to the posterior superior iliac spine, toward the top of the greater trochanter, and its lower border runs from the ischial tuberosity to a point ~ 10–15 cm inferior to the greater trochanter.

Gluteus medius and minimus These sit over the posterolateral and lateral surface of the hip bone, in the depression superolateral to gluteus maximus. Gluteus minimus sits deep to medius. Both attach to the greater trochanter. Weakness or paralysis leads to pelvic tilt toward the unsupported (contralateral) side when standing on one leg (Trendelenburg's sign).

Lateral rotator muscle group This group sits deep to gluteus maximus. The upper muscles overlie the hip joint and can be used to landmark its position. They are reflected medially during posterior surgical approaches to the hip.
- **Piriformis** passes along a line joining the greater trochanter to a point two fifths of the way down the line between the

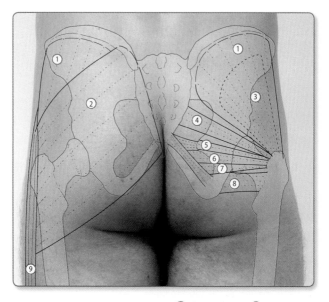

Figure 5.8 Muscles of the gluteal region. ① Gluteus medius, ② gluteus maximus, ③ gluteus minimus, ④ piriformis, ⑤ superior gemellus, ⑥ obturator internus, ⑦ inferior gemellus , ⑧ quadratus femoris, ⑨ iliotibial band/tract.

posterior superior iliac spine and ischial tuberosity. It marks the level of the sacral plexus (located anteriorly) and can be the source of gluteal region pain or sciatic nerve compression
- **Obturator internus** passes along a line joining a point ~ 5 cm superior to the ischial tuberosity to the top of the greater trochanter. It is flanked by gemellus superior and inferior
- **Quadratus femoris** passes from the ischial tuberosity to just below the greater trochanter

Posterior compartment
The hamstring muscle group This group is best seen whilst flexing the knee against resistance (**Figure 5.9**). Proximally the three muscles originate from the ischial tuberosity.

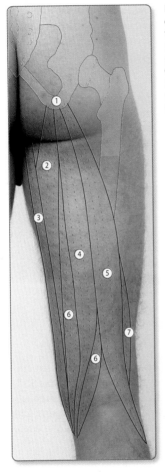

Figure 5.9 Posterior thigh compartment muscles. ① Ischial tuberosity, ② adductor magnus (medial compartment), ③ gracilis (medial compartment), ④ semitendinosus, ⑤ long head of biceps femoris, ⑥ semi-membranosus, ⑦ short head of biceps femoris.

- **Semitendinosus** and **semimembranosus** pass inferiorly along the medial side of the posterior thigh and can be palpated passing inferomedially across the knee to the tibia. Both contribute to the musculotendinous mass that passes over the medial knee

- **Biceps femoris** (long head) passes inferolaterally through the posterior thigh and is joined by the short head distally. The biceps tendon can be palpated passing inferolaterally over the lateral knee to the fibula head

Medial compartment

Adductor muscle group This group forms the muscle mass on the medial and anteromedial thigh (**Figure 5.10**). They pass from the pubis and ischial tuberosity to the femoral shaft and tibia. The group consists of four muscles:

- **Adductor longus** passes from the pubis to the middle third of the femoral shaft. It forms the prominent tendon that can be palpated in the groin region, especially during resisted limb adduction
- **Adductor magnus** passes inferolaterally from the ischial tuberosity to most of the posteromedial femoral shaft. Inferiorly its tendon can be palpated between vastus medialis and sartorius as it joins the adductor tubercle
- **Adductor brevis** passes inferolaterally from the pubis to the upper third of the femoral shaft
- **Gracilis** passes inferiorly along the medial thigh from the pubis to the proximal medial tibia

Anterior compartment

Tensor fascia lata This is seen and palpated passing posteroinferiorly from the anterior iliac crest to the iliotibial band (**Figure 5.11**). The anterior surgical approach to the hip (Smith Petersen) utilises the interval between tensor fascia lata and sartorius. Care needs to be taken during this approach to identify the lateral cutaneous nerve of the thigh.

Sartorius This passes inferomedially across the anterior thigh from the anterior superior iliac spine to the midpoint of the medial thigh from where it passes inferiorly to the tibia. It marks the position of the femoral artery and nerve in the midthigh region.

Quadriceps group This group consists of four muscles, which are best seen whilst seated with the knee extended and the hip flexed against resistance. The three vastus muscles originate

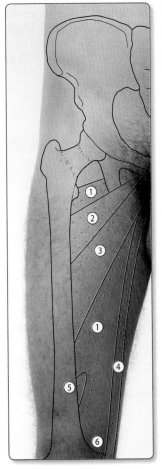

Figure 5.10 Medial thigh compartment muscles. ① Adductor magnus, ② adductor brevis, ③ adductor longus, ④ gracilis, ⑤ adductor hiatus (for femoral artery), ⑥ adductor tubercle.

from the femur, and rectus femoris from the anterior inferior iliac spine. All converge on the quadriceps tendon and patella.

- **Rectus femoris** is the wide band of muscle passing along a line from the anterior superior iliac spine to the patellar base. Rupture of its muscle belly causes thigh pain and a palpable/visible sulcus

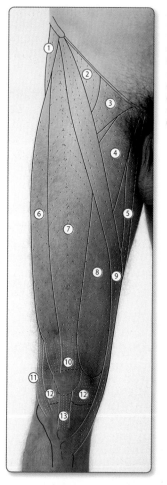

Figure 5.11 Anterior thigh compartment muscles. ① Tensor fascia lata, ② iliopsoas, ③ pectineus, ④ adductor longus, ⑤ gracilis, ⑥ vastus lateralis, ⑦ rectus femoris (overlying vastus intermedius), ⑧ vastus medialis, ⑨ sartorius, ⑩ quadriceps tendon, ⑪ iliotibial tract/band, ⑫ patellar retinacula, ⑬ patellar ligament.

- **Vastus intermedius** sits deep to rectus femoris and follows a similar course
- **Vastus lateralis** passes down the anterolateral thigh. It is covered and flattened by the iliotibial tract and ends as a curved prominence proximal to the patella base. Vastus

lateralis and the overlying iliotibial band can be incised to access the femoral shaft

- **Vastus medialis** forms the prominent muscle mass on the lower anteromedial thigh. It ends in a curve at the level of the patellar base

Patellar ligament This connects the apex of the patella to the prominent tibial tubercle. Tapping the ligament tests the L2-3 reflex. In anterior fat pad syndrome, the infrapatella fat pad, sat deep to the ligament, can become trapped and inflamed, resulting in intermittent anterior knee pain and a clicking sound on motion (**Figure 5.12**).

Bursae

Synovial bursae are found at multiple points of wear in the lower limb. Inflammation can lead to localised pain and swelling and require local steroid injection (**Table 5.3** and **Figures 5.13** and **5.14**).

Femoral triangle

The femoral triangle is located in the proximal anterior thigh (**Figure 5.15**). It is bordered:

Clinical insight

Knee joint injection or aspiration takes place via site 1 cm superior and 1 cm lateral to the superolateral patellar border, into the suprapatellar bursa.

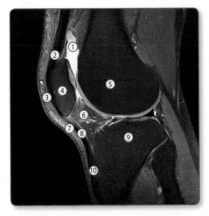

Figure 5.12 Sagittal MRI of the knee. (1) Suprapatellar bursa, (2) quadriceps tendon, (3) prepatellar bursa, (4) patella, (5) femoral condyle, (6) infrapatellar fat pad, (7) superficial part of infrapatellar bursa, (8) patellar ligament, (9) tibial condyle, (10) tibial tuberosity.

Bursa	Surface markings	Bursitis symptoms
Trochanteric	Superficial to the greater trochanter	Tenderness to palpation or on walking
Ischial	Inferior to the ischial tuberosity	Tenderness to palpation or on sitting
Anserine	Deep to the pes anserinus* over the medial proximal tibia	Medial knee pain on use and tenderness to palpation
Prepatellar	Anterior to the patella	Presents as painful anterior patellar swelling (Housemaid's knee)
Infrapatellar	Superficial and deep to the patellar ligament	Presents as a swelling around the patellar ligament (Clergyman's knee)
Suprapatellar	Extension of the knee-joint cavity that extends several centimetres above the patella in the midline	Knee joint effusion causes suprapatellar swelling. Inferiorly squeezing/milking a swollen bursa can produce a positive patellar tap test

*The pes anserineus is formed by sartorius, gracilis and semitendinosus attaching to the medial tibial condyle.

Table 5.3 Bursa of the gluteal region, thigh and knee.

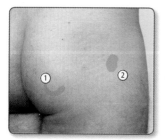

Figure 5.13 Gluteal and hip region bursae: posterolateral view. ① Ischial bursa ② trochanteric bursa.

- Superiorly by the inguinal ligament
- Laterally by the medial border of sartorius
- Medially by the lateral border of adductor longus

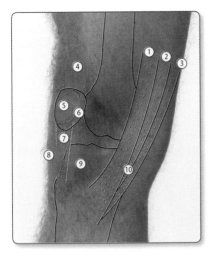

Figure 5.14 Bursae of the right knee and the pes anserinus: antero-medial view. ① Sartorius, ② gracilis, ③ semitendinosus, ④ suprapatellar bursa (deep to quadriceps tendon), ⑤ prepatellar bursa, ⑥ patella, ⑦ patellar ligament, ⑧ infrapatellar bursa: superficial part, ⑨ infrapatellar bursa: deep part, ⑩ anserine bursa (sat deep to pes anserinus).

- Anteriorly (roof) by fascia lata
- Posteriorly (floor) by iliopsoas, pectineus and adductor brevis

The femoral triangle contains, or is related to, the structures listed in **Table 5.4**.

Femoral sheath, canal, ring and hernias

The femoral sheath is an extension of the extraperitoneal fascia that covers the proximal 3 cm of the femoral artery, vein and lymphatics. It binds to the artery and vein but not to the lymphatics thus forming a channel, the femoral canal, through which hernias can pass. Femoral hernias enter the canal via the femoral ring, which sits posterior to the inguinal ligament ~ 1.5 cm lateral to the pubic tubercle. Small femoral hernias present as swellings lateral and inferior to the pubic tubercle whereas larger hernias pass through the saphenous opening and are reflected superiorly over the inguinal ligament.

Clinical insight

The timing of the femoral pulse can be delayed compared to the radial in aortic coarctation, or its volume reduced in iliac or aortic disease.

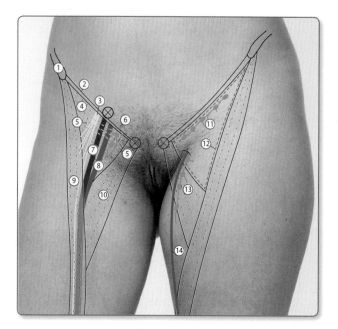

Figure 5.15 Femoral triangle. ① Anterior superior iliac spine, ② inguinal ligament, ③ femoral nerve, ④ iliopsoas, ⑤ femoral sheath (grey hatch), ⑥ deep inguinal lymph nodes (Cloquet's node in femoral canal), ⑦ femoral artery, ⑧ femoral vein, ⑨ sartorius and subsartorial/adductor canal, ⑩ adductor longus, ⑪ superficial inguinal lymph nodes (proximal group), ⑫ femoral triangle border, ⑬ superficial inguinal lymph nodes (distal group), ⑭ long saphenous vein, ⊗ midinguinal point, ⊗ pubic tubercle.

Neurovascular

Femoral artery and vein

The femoral artery enters the anterior thigh at the midinguinal point, ± 1.5 cm either side (**Figures 5.15–5.17**). The femoral vein sits ~ 1 cm medial to the artery. Both vessels pass inferiorly to enter the adductor canal at the femoral triangle apex. The canal runs deep to sartorius down the distal two thirds of the medial thigh to the adductor hiatus, an opening in adductor magnus approximately two thirds of the way down the canal, where the

Structure	Surface markings
Femoral nerve	Sits ~ 1 cm lateral to the femoral artery. Can be anaesthetised in this location
Femoral artery	Posterior to the midinguinal point (± 1.5 cm medial-lateral) where its pulsations are felt. Cannulated here for angiography
Femoral vein	Sits ~ 1 cm medial to the femoral artery. Can be cannulated (medial to the pulsating artery) to access the right side of the heart
Deep inguinal lymph nodes	Sit medial to the femoral vein. A prominent node (Cloquet) is often felt near the inguinal ligament. Receive lymph from the limb, perineum and lower abdominal wall
Long saphenous vein	Passes superficially over the roof to enter the saphenous opening. Accompanied by the distal group of superficial inguinal lymph nodes, which receive lymph from the limb
Saphenous opening	Sits ~ 3–4 cm inferolateral to the pubic tubercle. Site for femoral hernia emergence and saphena varix (long saphenous vein varicosity), which can also present as a regional swelling/hernia
Profunda femoris artery	Branch of femoral artery arising ~ 3–5 cm inferior to the inguinal ligament
Superficial inguinal lymph nodes	Proximal group sit along the inferior border of the inguinal ligament and receive lymph from the abdominal wall, gluteal region and perineum

Table 5.4 Contents and relations of the femoral triangle.

vessels pass into the popliteal fossa. On an abducted laterally rotated limb the femoral vessels can be mapped along the upper three quarters of a line passing from the midinguinal point to the adductor tubercle (**Figure 5.17**).

Profunda femoris artery This artery branches from the lateral side of the femoral artery ~ 3–5 cm inferior to the inguinal ligament (**Figure 5.16**). It gives rise to medial and lateral femoral circumflex arteries ~ 1–2 cm distal to its origin then

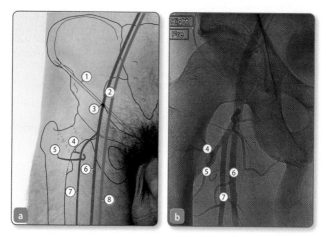

Figure 5.16 Femoral artery and its branches in the right anterior thigh. (a) Surface anatomy. (b) Arteriogram of the hip. ① Inguinal ligament, ② external iliac artery and vein, ③ midinguinal point, ④ medial circumflex femoral artery, ⑤ lateral circumflex femoral artery, ⑥ femoral artery, ⑦ profunda femoris artery, ⑧ femoral vein.

passes inferiorly along the medial femoral shaft where it can be identified on arteriograms.

Femoral nerve

The femoral nerve enters the femoral triangle 1 cm lateral to the pulsating femoral artery (**Figure 5.17**). Its saphenous branch accompanies the femoral artery and vein deep to sartorius, but continues inferomedially to pass onto the medial aspect of the knee from where it passes distally with the long saphenous vein.

Obturator nerve

The obturator nerve passes inferiorly through the obturator canal, located ~ 2 cm lateral and 2 cm inferior to the pubic tubercle, into the medial compartment. It can be anaesthetised as it passes out of the obturator canal or compressed via instrumentation placed deep to transverse acetabular ligament during hip surgery.

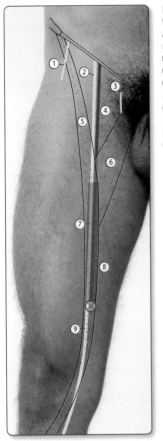

Figure 5.17 Neurovasculature of the antero-medial right thigh and adductor canal. ① Lateral cutaneous nerve of the thigh, ② femoral nerve, ③ obturator nerve, ④ femoral artery, ⑤ sartorius, ⑥ adductor longus, ⑦ saphenous nerve and femoral artery in adductor/subsartorial canal, ⑧ region of adductor/subsartorial canal (blue), ⑨ saphenous nerve, Ⓧ position of adductor hiatus, Ⓧ pubic tubercle.

Lateral cutaneous nerve of thigh

Passes inferiorly, deep to the inguinal ligament and inferome-dial to the anterior superior iliac spine where it can become trapped by tight clothing or overhanging abdominal fat causing lateral thigh paraesthesia. The nerve can be damaged during anterior (Smith Petersen) surgical approaches to the hip and can be anaesthetised via a site 2 cm inferior and 2 cm medial to the anterior superior iliac spine.

Sciatic nerve

The sciatic nerve enters the gluteal region via the greater sciatic foramen (infrapiriform part) and curves inferolaterally over the lateral rotators into the posterior thigh where it passes inferiorly, deep to biceps femoris (**Figure 5.18**). It bifurcates into the tibial and common fibular nerves approximately two thirds of the way down the thigh, near the superior apex of the popliteal fossa. The sciatic nerve can be traced between the following points and anaesthetised within the gluteal region:

- Midpoint of a line joining the posterior superior iliac spine to the ischial tuberosity
- The midpoint or middle third of a line joining the ischial tuberosity to the upper greater trochanter
- Midpoint of the long head of biceps femoris

Posterior cutaneous nerve of the thigh

This emerges from the infrapiriform part of the greater sciatic foramen and passes inferiorly between the long head of biceps femoris and the fascia lata. Distally it travels over the popliteal fossa to accompany the short saphenous vein in the proximal leg.

5.2 Knee, popliteal fossa and leg

Bones, joints and ligaments

Tibia

The tibia passes between the knee and ankle (**Figure 5.19**). Many features are palpable and can be used to landmark underlying structures.

- The **medial** and **lateral tibial condyles** are palpable around the knee margins, inferior to the femoral condyles
- The **tibial tuberosity** sits in line with the patellar ligament, ~ 3–5 cm inferior to the knee joint line. Pain over the

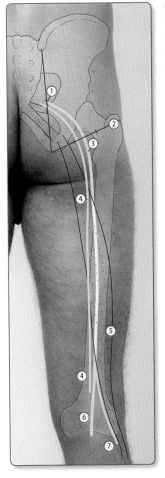

Figure 5.18 Course of the sciatic nerve in the gluteal region and posterior right thigh. ① Position of infrapiriform part of greater sciatic foramen, ② greater trochanter–ischial tuberosity line (divided into thirds), ③ sciatic nerve, ④ posterior cutaneous nerve of the thigh, ⑤ long head of biceps femoris, ⑥ tibial nerve, ⑦ common fibular nerve.

tuberosity can indicate avulsion fracture or Osgood–Schlatter lesion in young patients
- **Gerdy's tubercle** is located ~ 1 cm distal to the knee joint line and ~ 2–3 cm lateral to the tibial tuberosity. Regional pain can indicate iliotibial band syndrome or avulsion fracture

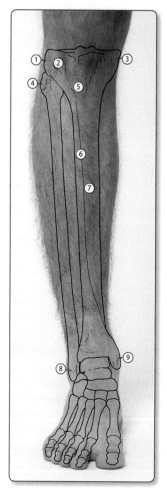

Figure 5.19 Anterior view of the bones of the right leg. ① Lateral tibial condyle, ② Gerdy's tubercle, ③ medial tibial condyle, ④ fibular head, ⑤ tibial tuberosity, ⑥ anterior border of tibia, ⑦ medial border of tibia, ⑧ lateral malleolus, ⑨ medial malleolus.

- The **medial tibial border** (shin) faces anteromedially and is fully palpable. It is continuous with the medial tibial condyle superiorly and the medial malleolus inferiorly

Fibula

The fibula passes down the lateral leg. It forms an articular surface of the ankle, but not the knee.

- **The fibula head** forms the rounded prominence palpated on the posterior region of the lateral leg ~ 1.5 cm inferior to the knee joint line
- **The biceps femoris tendon** can be traced inferiorly to the fibula head and the common fibular nerve sits immediately inferior to the tendon, where it can be damaged
- **The shaft** is palpable distally where it is continuous with the lateral malleolus

Knee joint

The lateral and medial femoral condyles are palpable either side of the patella and with the knee flexed their curved articular surface can be palpated (**Figure 5.20**). The medial-to-lateral knee joint line sits parallel to the ground and can be palpated as a near horizontal groove between the femoral and tibial condyles. The horizontal skin crease over the popliteal fossa sits ~ 2 cm proximal to the knee joint line. Arthroscopy ports can be made over the joint line either side of the patellar ligament.

Menisci The fibrocartilagenous menisci encircle the medial and lateral tibial condyles. Their outer margins can be palpated anteriorly either side of the patella at the knee joint line (**Figure 5.20**). Meniscal tearing from trauma, twisting and age-related degeneration can cause knee pain, locking or catching during motion, joint line tenderness and effusion.

Tendons crossing the knee Several tendons can be identified crossing the knee when it is flexed to 90° and resisting extension (**Table 5.5** and **Figures 5.21** and **5.22**).

Ligaments Strong ligaments support the knee joint laterally and medially (**Figures 5.21** and **5.22**).

Clinical insight

The tendons of gracilis and semitendinosus are often used for anterior cruciate ligament reconstruction.

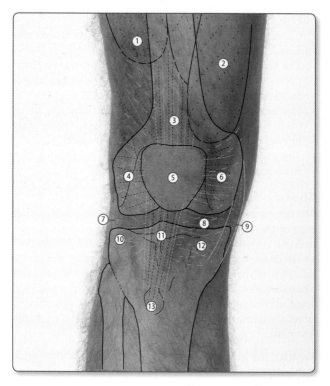

Figure 5.20 Anterior view of the right knee. (1) Vastus lateralis, (2) vastus medialis, (3) quadriceps tendon, (4) lateral femoral condyle, (5) patella, (6) medial femoral condyle, (7) lateral meniscus, (8) medial meniscus, (9) medial (tibial) collateral ligament, (10) lateral tibial condyle, (11) patellar ligament, (12) medial tibial condyle, (13) tibial tuberosity.

- The **lateral (fibular) collateral ligament** is a round cord that passes between the lateral femoral epicondyle and the fibular head. It is best palpated proximal to the fibula head, with laterally directed (varus) force applied to the medial knee. Excess varus forces can damage the ligament
- The **medial (tibial) collateral ligament** is a flattened band that passes between the medial femoral epicondyle,

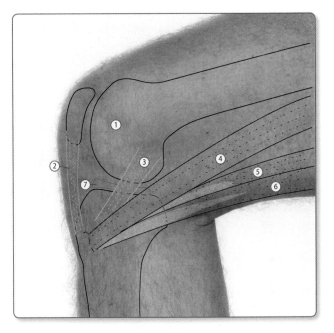

Figure 5.21 Medial view of the right knee. (1) Medial femoral condyle, (2) patellar ligament, (3) medial (tibial) collateral ligament, (4) sartorius, (5) gracilis and tendon, (6) semitendinosus and tendon, (7) medial meniscus.

Medial aspect	Lateral aspect
Semitendinosus distinct posterolaterally located tendon	**Biceps femoris** distinct posterolaterally located tendon
Gracilis distinct tendon located anteromedially to semitendinosus	**Iliotibial tract** firm broad band passing over the lateral condyles
Sartorius soft mass located anterior to gracilis	

Table 5.5 Tendons crossing the lateral and medial knee.

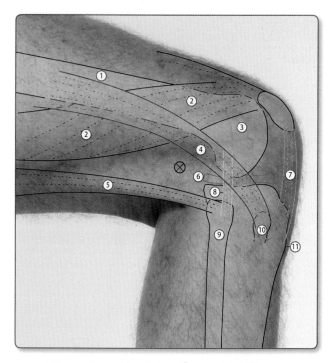

Figure 5.22 Lateral view of the right knee. ① Femoral shaft, ② vastus lateralis, ③ lateral femoral condyle, ④ iliotibial tract/band, ⑤ biceps femoris, ⑥ lateral meniscus, ⑦ patellar ligament, ⑧ lateral (fibular) collateral ligament, ⑨ fibular head and neck, ⑩ Gerdy's tubercle, ⑪ tibial tuberosity, ⊗ needle insertion point for tibial and common fibular nerve block.

the medial surface of the proximal tibia and the medial meniscus. Excess medially directed (valgus) force can damage both the ligament and medial meniscus

Muscles, tendons and regions
Posterior compartment
Gastrocnemius and soleus These are large and superficial (**Figure 5.23**). Both converge on the broad calcaneal (Achilles) tendon, which can be seen passing inferiorly and attaching

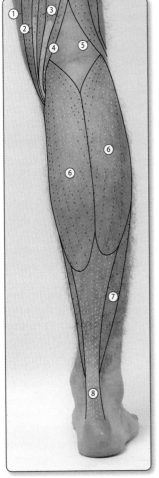

Figure 5.23 Posterior knee and superficial muscles of the posterior compartment. (1) Sartorius, (2) gracilis tendon, (3) semimembranosus, (4) semitendinosus, (5) biceps femoris, (6) gastrocnemius, (7) soleus, (8) tendocalcaneus/Achilles' tendon.

to the posterior surface of calcaneus. Retrocalcaneal bursitis presents as tenderness anterior to the tendon. Tapping the tendon tests

Clinical insight

Achilles tendon rupture can present with sudden sharp pain, functional loss, a round lump over the rupture and tenderness on palpation.

the S1–2 reflex. A reduced reflex can indicate cauda equina syndrome or an L5–S1 disc prolapse.

- **Gastrocnemius** is the most superficial muscle of the posterior leg. Its lateral and medial heads attach to the respective femoral condyles and its two bellies pass inferiorly to around mid-leg level
- **Soleus** sits deep to gastrocnemius but can be seen bulging around its lateral and medial sides. It attaches to the posterior surface of the fibula head, the proximal third of the posterior fibular shaft and the tibial soleal line (**Figure 5.24**)

The deep posterior compartment muscles These pass posterior to the medial malleolus to access the plantar foot (**Figure 5.24**). Foot inversion aids tendon identification.

- **Tibialis posterior** passes inferomedially from the superior two thirds of the fibula, tibia and interosseous membrane. It passes immediately posterior to the medial malleolus
- **Flexor digitorum longus** passes inferiorly from the middle third of the posterior tibial shaft and its tendon passes posterolateral to tibialis posterior at the ankle. The pulsation of the tibial artery is palpable posterolateral to the tendon
- **Flexor hallucis longus** passes inferolaterally from the posterior of the middle third of the fibula and its tendon passes posterolateral to flexor digitorum longus at the ankle

Popliteal fossa

The popliteal fossa is the diamond-shaped indentation located posterior to the knee (**Figure 5.25**). It is bordered:

- Superolaterally by biceps femoris
- Superomedially by semitendinosus and semimembranosus
- Inferolaterally by the lateral head of gastrocnemius
- Inferomedially by the medial head of gastrocnemius

The fossa is fat filled and extends between the deep fascia of the limb and posterior femur/knee. The fossa contains or is related to the structures listed in **Table 5.6**.

The tibial and common fibular nerve can be anaesthetised in the fossa. The lateral approach enters the fossa via a point where the groove between biceps femoris and vastus lateralis

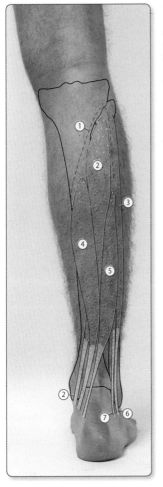

Figure 5.24 Deep muscles of the posterior compartment of the leg. ① Soleal arch, ② tibialis posterior, ③ lateral leg compartment, ④ flexor digitorum longus, ⑤ flexor hallucis longus, ⑥ fibularis longus, ⑦ fibularis brevis.

is intersected by a line drawn level with the patellar base (**Figure 5.22**). The posterior approach enters the fossa near its superior apex.

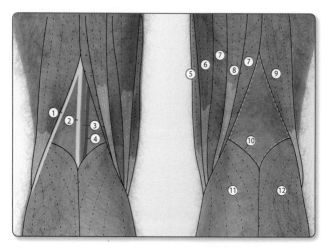

Figure 5.25 Popliteal fossae of the left and right knees (posterior view). ① Common fibular nerve, ② tibial nerve, ③ popliteal vein, ④ popliteal artery, ⑤ sartorius, ⑥ gracilis, ⑦ semimembranosus, ⑧ semitendinosus, ⑨ biceps femoris, ⑩ border of popliteal fossa, ⑪ medial head of gastrocnemius, ⑫ lateral head of gastrocnemius.

Structure	Surface markings
Popliteal artery	Passes inferiorly along the fossa floor; aneurysm produces a pulsatile swelling in the fossa; can be lacerated via supracondylar fracture
Popliteal vein	Passes inferiorly through the fossa, superficial and lateral to the popliteal artery
Tibial nerve	Passes inferiorly through the fossa, superficial and lateral to the popliteal vein; injury here causes loss of push-off (plantarflexion) during walking
Common fibular nerve	Passes inferolaterally along the lower border of biceps femoris to the lateral fibula neck; injury here causes foot drop

Table 5.6 Contents of the popliteal fossa.

Synovial cysts These cysts form non-pulsatile popliteal fossa swellings that can burst causing oedema or pain. Baker cysts connect with the knee-joint cavity and often present below the joint line level whereas popliteal cysts of the semimembranosus/ medial gastrocnemius bursae present medially and above the joint line level.

Anterior compartment

The anterior compartment muscles form a prominent mass in the upper two thirds of the anterolateral leg, especially noticeable during foot dorsiflexion (**Figure 5.26**). In athletes regional pain can be caused by medial tibial stress syndrome (shin splints), chronic exertional compartment syndrome or tibial stress fracture.

Tibialis anterior This passes inferomedially from the proximal half of the lateral tibia. Its prominent tendon can be seen and palpated as it crosses the ankle and medial foot to insert into the base of the 1st metatarsal and medial cuneiform.

Extensor hallucis longus This passes inferomedially from the middle of the fibula across the ankle to the great toe. The dorsalis pedis artery sits lateral to the tendon on the dorsal foot.

Extensor digitorum This passes inferiorly from the proximal three quarters of the anterior fibula and lateral tibial condyle. Its tendon can be palpated anterior to the ankle and on the dorsal foot as it divides into four and passes to digits 2–5.

Fibularis tertius This passes from the distal anterior fibula to the base of the 5th metatarsal. Its thin tendon is best palpated in foot eversion just anterior to the lateral malleolus.

Lateral compartment

Fibularis longus This passes inferiorly from the proximal half of the lateral fibula and posterior to the lateral malleolus (**Figure 5.27**). Foot eversion enables palpation of its tendon

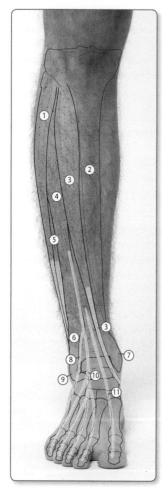

Figure 5.26 Muscles of the anterior and lateral compartments. (1) Fibularis longus, (2) medial tibial border, (3) tibialis anterior, (4) extensor digitorum longus, (5) fibularis brevis, (6) distal fibula, (7) medial malleolus, (8) tendon of fibularis tertius, (9) lateral malleolus, (10) extensor digitorum longus dividing into 4 tendons, (11) tendon of extensor hallucis longus.

posterior to the lateral malleolus. The posterolateral surgical approach to the tibia and fibula is via an incision between fibularis longus and soleus.

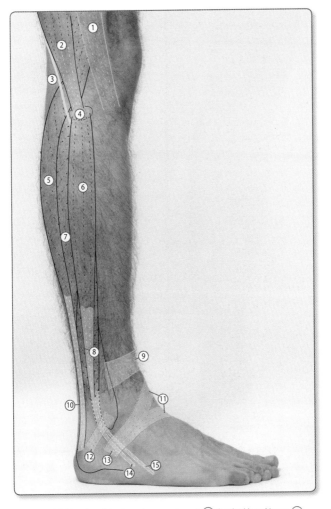

Figure 5.27 Muscles of the lateral compartment. (1) Iliotibial band/tract, (2) biceps femoris, (3) common fibular nerve, (4) fibular head, (5) gastrocnemius, (6) fibularis longus, (7) soleus, (8) fibularis brevis, (9) superior extensor retinaculum, (10) Achilles tendon, (11) inferior extensor retinaculum, (12) superior fibular retinaculum, (13) inferior fibular retinaculum, (14) fibularis longus tendon, (15) fibularis brevis tendon.

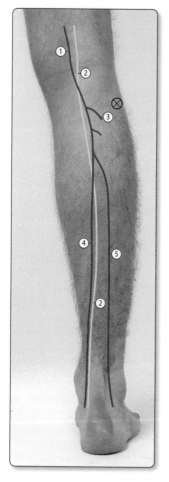

Figure 5.28 Neurovasculature of the posterior compartment. ① Popliteal artery, ② tibial nerve, ③ anterior tibial artery passing to anterior compartment, ④ posterior tibial artery, ⑤ fibular artery, Ⓧ fibular head.

Fibularis brevis This passes inferiorly from the middle half of the lateral fibula and posterior to the lateral malleolus. Its tendon can be palpated during foot eversion as it passes from behind the lateral malleolus to the 5th metatarsal tuberosity. Tendon avulsion can occur from excessive foot inversion.

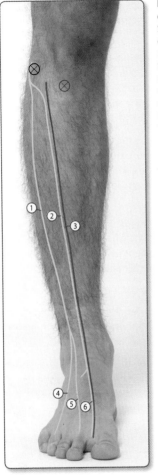

Figure 5.29 Neurovasculature of the anterior compartment. ① Superficial fibular nerve (lateral compartment), ② deep fibular nerve (anterior compartment), ③ anterior tibial artery, ④ intermediate dorsal cutaneous nerve, ⑤ medial dorsal cutaneous nerve, ⑥ medial branch of deep fibular nerve and dorsalis pedis artery, ⊗ fibular head, ⊗ tibial tuberosity.

Neurovasculature

Arteries

Popliteal artery and branches The popliteal artery passes inferiorly through the popliteal fossa close to the femur against which its pulsation can be palpated and it can be lacerated via distal femoral fracture (**Figure 5.28** and **5.29**). It passes deep to soleus and bifurcates level with the lower part of the fibula head/tibial tuberosity.

Posterior tibial artery This passes inferiorly through the posterior compartment (anterior to soleus) along a line joining a point midway between the tibial condyles to a point one third of the way along a line joining the medial malleolus to the Achilles tendon where it enters the tarsal tunnel.

Anterior tibial artery This enters the anterior compartment at a point midway between the palpable fibula head and tibial tuberosity and passes inferiorly to a point midway between the malleoli, where it sits lateral to extensor hallucis longus.

Fibular artery This artery branches off the posterior tibial ~ 8–10 cm inferior to the knee joint line and passes inferiorly through the posterior compartment just medial to the fibula and onto the posterior of the lateral malleolus.

Nerves

Tibial nerve This nerve passes inferiorly along the midline of the popliteal fossa and through the posterior leg where it is landmarked with the posterior tibial artery.

Common fibular nerve This nerve passes inferolaterally with the biceps femoris tendon and then curves around the lateral fibula neck, where it can be palpated as a firm cord and is vulnerable to compression/injury. It then travels deep to fibularis longus where it bifurcates:

- The **superficial fibular nerve** passes inferiorly deep to fibularis longus. It emerges two thirds of the way down the anterolateral fibula and branches into the medial and intermediate dorsal cutaneous nerves, which travel on to the dorsal foot
- The **deep fibular nerve** travels inferiorly with the anterior tibial artery on to the dorsal foot and its medial branch passes to the web space between digits 1 and 2.

Superficial veins and cutaneous nerves

The saphenous veins originate from the dorsal venous arch of the foot and pass close to the malleoli, where they can be accessed in emergencies via an incision/venous cutdown (**Table 5.7** and **Figures 5.30** and **5.31**). Cutaneous nerves sit close to the veins distally and can be anaesthetised near the malleoli or damaged during varicose vein removal.

Infrapatellar nerves The infrapatellar nerves branch off the saphenous nerves around the level of the apex of the patella and curve around to the patella and its ligament (**Figure 5.30**). They can be damaged during knee arthroscopy or an anteromedial surgical approach, which can cause persistent anterior knee pain.

5.3 Ankle and foot

Bones, joints and ligaments
Bones of the foot

Many features of the bones and joints of the foot can be identified on the dorsum or sides of the foot via palpation (**Table 5.8**

Vein	Origin and surface markings	Associated nerve
Short (small) saphenous	Passes posterior to the lateral malleolus and ascends the midline of the posterior leg to the popliteal fossa	Sural cutaneous nerve in the posterior leg and lateral foot
Long (great) saphenous	Passes anterior to the medial malleolus, ascends the medial tibia and passes over the medial femoral condyle ~ 7 cm posterior to the patella. Ascends the anteromedial thigh to the saphenous opening (~ 3–4 cm inferolateral to the pubic tubercle)	Saphenous nerve in the medial leg and dorsomedial foot; cutaneous branches of obturator/femoral nerve in the medial thigh

Table 5.7 Saphenous (superficial) veins and cutaneous nerves.

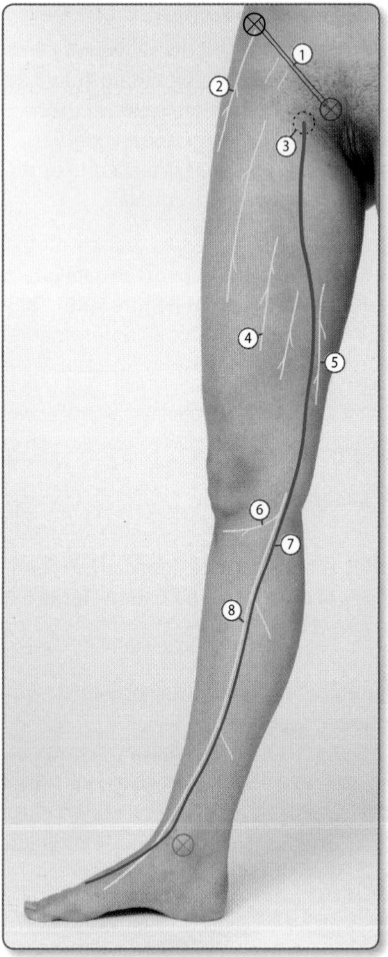

Figure 5.30 Long saphenous vein and cutaneous nerves of the lower limb. (1) Inguinal ligament, (2) lateral cutaneous nerve of the thigh, (3) saphenous opening and long saphenous vein, (4) anterior cutaneous nerves (femoral branches), (5) cutaneous branch of obturator nerve, (6) infrapatellar nerve, (7) long saphenous vein, (8) saphenous nerve, (X) anterior superior iliac spine, (X) pubic tubercle, (X) medial malleolus.

and **Figures 5.32** and **5.33**). Fractures are common and can be accompanied by pain that increases with motion, inability to weight bear, swelling, local bruising and deformity.

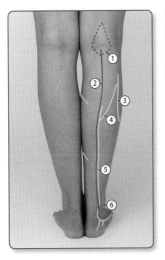

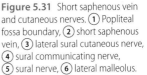

Figure 5.31 Short saphenous vein and cutaneous nerves. ① Popliteal fossa boundary, ② short saphenous vein, ③ lateral sural cutaneous nerve, ④ sural communicating nerve, ⑤ sural nerve, ⑥ lateral malleolus.

Metatarsals, phalanges and joints The long metatarsal bodies can be traced to the expanded heads, which articulate with the proximal phalanx at the metatarsophalangeal joint. The metatarsophalangeal joint line is easily palpated on the dorsal foot and can be injected/aspirated via this approach. The phalanges and interphalangeal joints are also easily palpated, with the joint line sitting proximal to the widest part of the joint. A valgus deformity of the 1st metatarsophalangeal joint (hallux valgus) is common and can be accompanied by a bunion, an inflamed bursa over the deformed joint.

Clinical insight

The spine must be checked for injury following a fall/jump onto the heel that fractures calcaneus.

Bones of the ankle

The ankle is formed between the distal tibia, medial malleolus, lateral malleolus and the talus. The inferior tip of the lateral malleolus normally sits more inferior and posterior than that of the medial malleolus. Alterations to this arrangement

Feature	Surface marking
Calcaneal tuberosity and processes	The tuberosity forms the main bony prominence of the heel. The processes sit either side and are the site of pain in plantar fasciitis
Fibula trochlea	Sits ~ 2 cm anteroinferior to the lateral malleolus. A point for fibularis tendon wear
Sustentaculum tali	Bony shelf sat ~ 2 cm inferior to the medial malleolus. Flexor hallucis longus passes inferiorly
Navicular tuberosity	Bony prominence that is seen and palpated ~ 2–3 cm anterior to the sustentaculum tali
Head of talus	Rounded prominence sat distal to the tibia and lateral to the extensor hallucis longus tendon on the dorsal foot. Foot inversion aids identification. Regional tenderness can indicate a talar neck fracture
Tuberosity of the 5th metatarsal base	Prominent posterolaterally pointing bony prominence. Subject to avulsion fracture following forced or excess ankle inversion
Transverse tarsal joint	Coronally-oriented joint line; can be identified anterior to the head of talus
Tarsometatarsal (Lisfranc) joint line	Bony ridge passing over the dorsal foot from a point ~ 2–3 cm anterior to the navicular tuberosity toward the tuberosity of the 5th metatarsal base. Can dislocate following high force injury

Table 5.8 Tarsal bones and joints of the foot.

suggest pathology. Palpation proximal to the talar head and neck reveals the ankle joint line and distal tibia. The joint can be injected/aspirated via the soft indented region between the medial malleolus and tibialis anterior.

Ligaments

Calcaneonavicular (spring) ligament The spring ligament passes between the sustentaculum tali and navicular tuberosity, where it is palpated as a firm band during foot eversion. Rupture can lead to localised pain, swelling and a flattened foot.

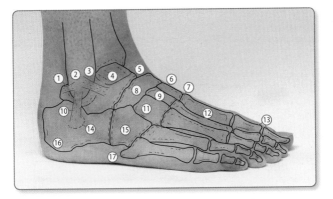

Figure 5.32 Lateral view of bones and ligaments of the foot. ① Posterior talofibular ligament, ② lateral malleolus, ③ anterior talofibular ligament, ④ trochlea of talus, ⑤ head of talus and transverse tarsal joint line (orange), ⑥ medial cuneiform, ⑦ tarsometatarsal joint line (orange), ⑧ navicular, ⑨ intermediate cuneiform, ⑩ calcaneofibular ligament, ⑪ lateral cuneiform, ⑫ 1st metatarsal, ⑬ phalanges of digit 1 (proximal and distal), ⑭ fibular trochlea, ⑮ cuboid, ⑯ calcaneal tuberosity, ⑰ tuberosity of 5th metatarsal. **Note:** ligaments 1, 3 and 10 collectively form the lateral collateral ligament.

Ankle ligaments The ligaments of the medial and lateral ankle are named and can be landmarked according to their attachments (**Figures 5.32** and **5.33**). The medial group collectively form the deltoid ligament. Regional injury is common. The ligaments are subject to sprains, especially the lateral, and can avulse the malleoli resulting in swelling, pain and inability to bear weight.

Muscles and tendons
Retinacula of the ankle
These are formed by thickenings of deep fascia (**Figures 5.34** and **5.35**). Retinacula tears cause pain, tendon bowstringing and malalignment. The tendons passing under the retinacula are covered by synovial sheaths, most of which extend from the distal leg into the foot and can act as routes for infection spread or can become inflamed in synovitis/tenosynovitis causing pain on use.

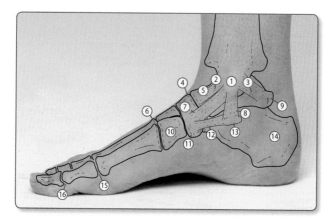

Figure 5.33 Bones and ligaments of the medial right foot. ① Medial malleolus, ② anterior tibiotalar ligament, ③ posterior tibiotalar ligament, ④ transverse tarsal joint line (orange), ⑤ head of talus, ⑥ tarsometatarsal joint line (orange), ⑦ tibionavicular ligament, ⑧ tibiocalcaneal ligament, ⑨ posterior process of talus, ⑩ medial cuneiform, ⑪ navicular tuberosity, ⑫ calcaneonavicular/spring ligament, ⑬ sustentaculum tali, ⑭ calcaneus, ⑮ first metatarsophalangeal joint, ⑯ interphalangeal joint of digit 1.
Note: ligaments 2, 3, 7 and 8 collectively form the medial collateral (deltoid) ligament.

- The **superior extensor retinaculum** passes from the distal fibula shaft to the distal tibia, a few centimetres proximal to the malleoli
- The **inferior extensor retinaculum** (Y-shaped) attaches laterally to calcaneus and bifurcates as it passes medially to attach to the medial malleolus and the navicular tuberosity
- The **flexor retinaculum** passes posteroinferiorly from the medial malleolus to the medial surface of calcaneus. It forms the roof of the tarsal tunnel where the tibial nerve can be compressed
- The **superior fibular retinaculum** passes posteroinferiorly between the lateral malleolus and calcaneus and the **inferior fibular retinaculum** between the inferior extensor retinaculum and calcaneus

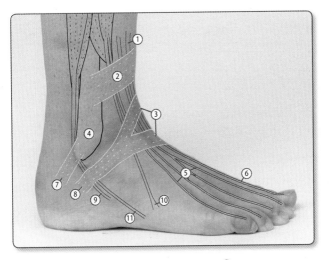

Figure 5.34 Tendons and retinacula of the lateral foot. ① Tibialis anterior, ② superior extensor retinaculum, ③ inferior extensor retinaculum, ④ lateral malleolus, ⑤ extensor digitorum longus, ⑥ extensor hallucis longus, ⑦ superior fibular retinaculum, ⑧ inferior fibular retinaculum, ⑨ fibularis longus tendon, ⑩ fibularis tertius, ⑪ fibularis brevis tendon attaching to tuberosity of 5th metatarsal.

Tarsal tunnel

The fibro-osseous tarsal tunnel is located posteroinferior to the medial malleolus between calcaneus and the flexor retinaculum (**Figure 5.35**). Its entrance sits on a line joining the medial malleolus to the upper part of calcaneus. Regional fracture, trauma or tendon ganglion can compress the tibial nerve and cause tarsal tunnel syndrome characterised by plantar foot pain/paraesthesia, which is worse at night, and wasting of plantar foot muscles. The tunnel contains the structures listed in **Table 5.9**.

Dorsal ankle and foot

Long extensor muscle tendons These pass on to the dorsal foot and can be traced to the digits especially during resisted dorsiflexion (**Figure 5.36**). Anterolateral surgical approaches to

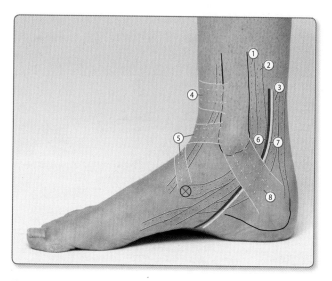

Figure 5.35 Tendons and retinacula of the medial right foot. ① Tibialis posterior, ② flexor digitorum longus, ③ flexor hallucis longus, ④ superior extensor retinaculum, ⑤ inferior extensor retinaculum, ⑥ posterior tibial artery, ⑦ tibial nerve, ⑧ flexor retinaculum covering tarsal tunnel, Ⓧ navicular tuberosity.

Structure	Surface markings and relevance
Tibialis posterior	Immediately behind the medial malleolus. Tendon rupture here or in the medial foot causes medial ankle and foot pain and a 2° flat foot
Flexor digitorum longus	Posterolateral to tibialis posterior
Posterior tibial artery	Sits posterior to flexor digitorum longus. Its pulsations are palpable here
Tibial nerve	Posterior to the tibial artery. Can be anaesthetised proximal to the tarsal tunnel
Flexor hallucis longus	The most posterolateral tendon in the tunnel. Tendonitis can present as pain and tenderness posterior to the medial malleolus

Table 5.9 Contents of the tarsal tunnel.

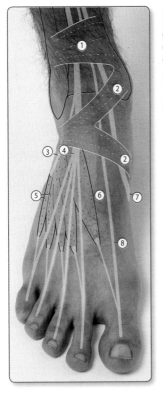

Figure 5.36 Extensor tendons and retinacula of the dorsal right foot. ① Superior extensor retinaculum, ② inferior extensor retinaculum, ③ fibularis tertius, ④ extensor digitorum longus, ⑤ extensor digitorum brevis, ⑥ extensor hallucis brevis, ⑦ tibialis anterior, ⑧ extensor hallucis longus.

the ankle pass between the extensor digitorum longus and the fibula. Tibialis anterior passes over the medial side of the foot to the base of the 1st metatarsal and the medial cuneiform.

Extensor digitorum brevis and extensor hallucis brevis These originate laterally from calcaneus where they can be palpated as a soft mass. Resisted digit dorsiflexion reveals tendons of the muscles travelling inferomedially to the proximal phalanges. Injury can produce an extensor compartment haematoma.

Plantar foot

Plantar aponeurosis The tough subcutaneous plantar aponeurosis passes from the calcaneal processes to each digit.
Repetitive high-impact activities can cause plantar fasciitis,
which presents with plantar foot and heel pain especially over
the medially calcaneal process. The pain is exacerbated by
passive dorsiflexion of great toe or ankle and can ease with
activity.

Intrinsic muscles and long flexor tendons The long flexor
tendons enter the foot posterolateral to the medial malleolus.
Flexor hallucis longus passes to digit 1 and flexor digitorum
longus to the base of metatarsal 2 or 3, where it divides into
four tendons that pass to digits 2–5. The intrinsic muscles on
the lateral and medial sides of the plantar foot are palpable.
The remainder sit deep to the retinaculum and are landmarked
by their attachments (**Table 5.10** and **Figures 5.37** and **5.38**).

Neurovasculature

Plantar arteries and nerves

The posterior tibial artery and tibial nerve bifurcate into the
medial and lateral plantar arteries and nerves ~ 1–2 cm inferior

Muscle	Surface markings
Abductor hallucis	Forms the fleshy muscle mass passing from the medial calcaneal process to the proximal phalanx of digit 1
Abductor digiti minimi	Forms the fleshy muscle mass passing from the lateral calcaneal processes to the proximal phalanx of digit 5
Flexor hallucis brevis and sesamoid bones	Passes along the 1st metatarsal to the proximal phalanx of digit 1. The sesamoid bones are palpable over the metatarsal head and can cause pain on walking/palpation following stress fracture or overuse (sesamoiditis)
Flexor digitorum brevis	Passes down the central foot from calcaneus to the middle phalanx of digits 2–5

Table 5.10 Intrinsic muscles of the plantar foot.

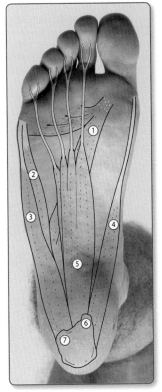

Figure 5.37 Intrinsic muscles of the plantar foot. (1) Adductor hallucis, (2) flexor digiti minimi brevis, (3) abductor digiti minimi, (4) abductor hallucis, (5) flexor digitorum brevis, (6) medial calcaneal process, (7) lateral calcaneal process.

to a point one third of the way along a line joining the medial malleolus to Achilles tendon. The arteries and nerves follow similar courses (**Figure 5.39**).

- The **lateral plantar branches** travel toward the middle of the 5th metatarsal, where the nerve sends digital branches along the sides of the lateral 1.5 digits and the artery curves medially across the proximal shaft of metatarsals 5–2 and gives off branches to the digits
- The **medial plantar branches** travel toward the base of the 1st metatarsal then send branches along the sides of the

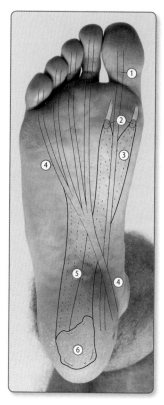

Figure 5.38 Intrinsic muscles and long flexor tendons of the plantar foot. ① Tendon of flexor hallucis longus, ② sesamoid bones of flexor hallucis brevis, ③ flexor hallucis brevis, ④ tendons of flexor digitorum longus, ⑤ quadratus plantae, ⑥ calcaneus.

medial 3.5 digits. Perineural fibrosis (Morton's neuroma) can affect the plantar digital nerve in the 3rd web space causing burning pain and digit numbness

Dorsal arteries and nerves

Dorsalis pedis artery and deep fibular nerve The dorsalis pedis artery passes onto the dorsal foot midway between the malleoli and lateral to the extensor hallucis longus tendon, where its pulsations are palpable. It passes distally toward the bases of metatarsals 1–2 at which point it curves laterally across

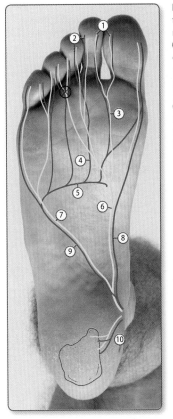

Figure 5.39 Neurovasculature of the plantar foot. ① Plantar digital nerves, ② plantar digital arteries, ③ common plantar nerve, ④ common plantar artery, ⑤ deep plantar arterial arch, ⑥ medial plantar nerve, ⑦ lateral plantar nerve, ⑧ medial plantar artery, ⑨ lateral plantar artery, ⑩ medial calcaneal artery and nerve, Ⓧ site of painful Morton's neuroma (perineural fibrosis).

the phalangeal bases as the arcuate artery (**Figure 5.40**). The deep fibular nerve travels alongside the dorsalis pedis artery. Its medial branch continues to the first web space, which it innervates. Its lateral branch arises distal to the inferior extensor retinaculum and passes laterally to innervate the dorsal intrinsic foot muscles.

Medial and intermediate cutaneous nerves The intermediate cutaneous nerve is seen and palpated as a fine ridge passing

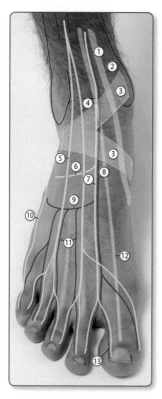

Figure 5.40 Neurovasculature of the dorsal foot. (1) Anterior tibial artery, (2) tibialis anterior tendon, (3) inferior extensor retinaculum, (4) medial dorsal cutaneous nerve, (5) intermediate dorsal cutaneous nerve, (6) lateral branch of deep fibular nerve, (7) medial branch of deep fibular nerve, (8) dorsalis pedis artery, (9) arcuate artery, (10) lateral dorsal cutaneous nerve, (11) dorsal metatarsal arteries, (12) extensor hallucis longus tendon, (13) dorsal digital arteries and nerves.

from the distal fibula toward digit 4 during foot and digit plantarflexion. It moves laterally by up to 5 mm when the foot is moved from plantarflexion to the neutral position and should be avoided during surgical approaches to the foot and ankle. The medial cutaneous nerve passes toward digit 2 but is not easily seen or palpated.

Digital arteries and nerves

The dorsal metatarsal arteries pass distally towards each of the web spaces and branch into digital arteries that travel along the sides of the digits alongside the digital sensory nerves.

A similar arrangement is seen on the plantar foot. The toes can therefore be anaesthetised using the same web space/ring block as the fingers (**Chapter 4**).

Pelvis and perineum

Pelvic region

The pelvic region is located at the inferior end of the abdominopelvic cavity. The term pelvis, pelvic cavity and pelvic girdle are often interchanged. Anatomical definitions of these terms are given in **Table 6.1**.

Perineum

The perineum is a diamond-shaped region located below the pelvic floor. It can be divided into urogenital and anal triangles. The urogenital triangle contains the external genitalia of both sexes and voluntary urinary sphincter muscles. The anal triangle contains the anal canal and the voluntary and autonomic anal sphincters. The lateral parts of the perineum also contain the fat-filled ischioanal fossae, which are prone to abscess and fistula formation.

Function

The pelvic girdle is adapted to permit bipedal locomotion and transmits forces between the vertebral column and lower limb. The pelvic cavity contains and protects multiple organs including

Feature/region	Definition
Pelvic girdle	Ring of bone formed by the hip bones and sacrum
Pelvis	Region bordered by the pelvic girdle. Subdivided into greater and lesser parts
Greater pelvis	Superiorly located region contained by the iliac fossa. Forms the lower part of the abdominal cavity
Lesser pelvis	Inferiorly located region contained by the bony walls of the pelvic cavity and perineum
Pelvic cavity	Region located within the lesser pelvis between the plane of the pelvic inlet and the pelvic floor muscles

Table 6.1 Definitions of pelvic structures and regions.

the rectum, bladder and ureters, in both sexes, and the uterus, uterine tubes, ovaries and vagina in the female and the prostate, seminal vesicles, and ductus deferens in the male.

6.1 Bones, joints and ligaments

The pelvic girdle is formed by the right and left hip bones and the sacrum. The hip bones are formed from three bones, the ilium, ischium and pubis, that fuse together during puberty (**Figures 6.1** and **6.2**). Many of the regional bony landmarks are shared with the abdomen, lower limb and back. They can easily be palpated and serve as landmarks for important planes and features.

Ilium

The ilium is located superiorly. Many of its features are palpable.

- The **iliac crest** is easily palpated from the anterior superior iliac spine to the posterior superior iliac spine

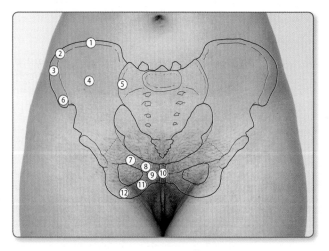

Figure 6.1 Bones of the anterior female pelvis. ① Highest point of iliac crest (supracristal plane), ② iliac crest, ③ tubercle of iliac crest, ④ iliac bone, ⑤ sacroiliac joint, ⑥ anterior superior iliac spine, ⑦ superior pubic ramus, ⑧ pubic tubercle, ⑨ body of pubis, ⑩ pubic symphysis, ⑪ inferior pubic ramus, ⑫ ischial tuberosity.

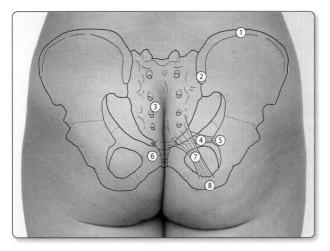

Figure 6.2 Bones and ligaments of the posterior female pelvis. ① Highest point of iliac crest (supracristal plane), ② posterior superior iliac spine, ③ sacrum, ④ sacrospinous ligament, ⑤ ischial spine, ⑥ coccyx, ⑦ sacrotuberous ligament, ⑧ ischial tuberosity.

- The **posterior superior iliac spine** marks the S2 vertebral level and the base of the sacral triangle, which is used as a landmark during caudal epidural
- The **anterior superior iliac spine** is the anteriormost projection of the iliac crest
- The **iliac tubercle** can be palpated 5–7 cm posterior to the anterior superior iliac spine and marks the L5 vertebral level
- The **highest point of the iliac crest** sits posteriorly and marks the L4 vertebral level (supracristal plane) during lumbar puncture

Ischium

The ischium is located posteroinferiorly. Many of its features are palpable.

- The **ramus** passes anterosuperiorly from the body to join with the inferior pubic ramus

- The **ischial tuberosity** is the curved most inferior section of bone of the pelvic girdle. It transmits the weight of the trunk when sitting and can be palpated lateral to the ischioanal fossa
- The **ischial spines** sit posterosuperior to the ischial tuberosities and project medially. They can be palpated during rectal or vaginal examination and mark the position of the pudendal nerve when anaesthetising the perineal region

> ### Clinical insight
>
> The ischial tuberosity is covered by a synovial bursa, which can become inflamed resulting in regional pain/tenderness on sitting or palpation.

Pubis
The pubis is located anteriorly and is easily palpated. Many of its features are palpable.
- The **body** sits either side of the midline pubic symphysis
- The **superior ramus** runs posterolaterally and connects to the ilium and ischium
- The **inferior ramus** runs inferolaterally and connects with the ischial ramus
- The **pubic tubercle** is a prominent landmark on the superior border of the body, located 2–3 cm from the midline. The superficial inguinal ring is located superolaterally

Ligaments
Sacrotuberous and sacrospinous ligaments
These ligaments connect the sacrum and coccyx to the ischium (**Figure 6.2**). They are useful landmarks for the positions of gluteal region structures (**Chapter 5**). Both can be palpated during digital rectal examination.
- The **sacrotuberous ligament** passes from the lower sacrum, coccyx and ilium to the posterior of the ischial tuberosity. In lean individuals it is palpable through the lower fibres of gluteus maximus
- The **sacrospinous ligament** passes from the lower part of the sacrum and coccyx to the ischial spine. It divides the sciatic foramen into greater and lesser parts and marks

the posterior level of the pelvic floor and laterally the position of the pudendal nerve (**Figure 6.21**), where it can be blocked

Joints

The two main joints of the pelvic girdle can be identified via the surface and on radiograph (**Figure 6.3**).

- The **pubic symphysis** is located anteriorly in the median sagittal plane between the bodies of the two pubic bones. It can be a source of regional pain, especially during late pregnancy
- The **sacroiliac joint** is located posteriorly between the sacrum and ilium, its midpoint sits deep to the posterior superior iliac spine. Pain from sacroiliac joint injury can refer to the gluteal region, perineum, iliac crest, perianal region, or the testicle, scrotum or penis in the male

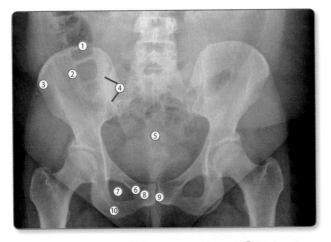

Figure 6.3 Pelvic radiograph. (1) Highest point of iliac crest, (2) iliac bone, (3) anterior superior iliac spine, (4) sacroiliac joint, (5) sacrum, (6) pubic tubercle, (7) obturator foramen, (8) pubic bone, (9) pubic symphysis, (10) ischial tuberosity.

Pelvic measurements

The lesser pelvis contributes to the birth canal of the female. The distances between specific features of the bones bordering the lesser pelvis are important in determining the ability to birth vaginally. Some can be measured via palpable features (**Table 6.2** and **Figures 6.4** and **6.5**).

Measurement	Description and measurement technique	Mean (cm)*
Intertuberous distance	Distance between the ischial tuberosities	12
Interspinous distance	Passes between the ischial spines; measured via vaginal examination	11
Diagonal conjugate	Passes from the sacral promontory to the outer surface of the pubic symphysis; measured via vaginal examination	12
True conjugate	Passes from sacral promontory to the inner superior surface of the pubic symphysis; estimated from diagonal conjugate minus 1.5 cm	10.5
*Measurements are variable between subjects.		

Table 6.2 Average female pelvic diameters.

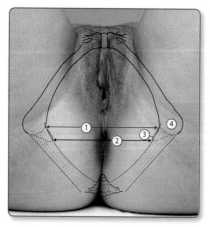

Figure 6.4 Female perineum: pelvic diameters.
① Intertuberous distance,
② interspinous distance,
③ ischial spine,
④ ischial tuberosity.

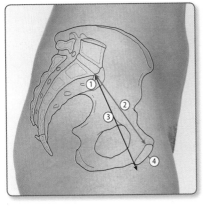

Figure 6.5 Lateral view of female pelvis: pelvic diameters. ① Sacral promontory, ② true conjugate, ③ diagonal conjugate, ④ pubic symphysis.

6.2 Perineum

Urogenital and anal triangles

The diamond-shaped perineum is located below the muscle of the pelvic floor and is bordered by the lower part of the pelvic girdle. A line drawn between the ischial tuberosities divides the region into a urogenital and an anal triangle (**Table 6.3** and **Figures 6.6** and **6.7**).

Triangle	Borders	Contents
Urogenital	Ischiopubic rami; pubic symphysis; intertuberous line	External genitalia; perineal membrane and pouches; urethra and external sphincter; bulbourethral gland (male); greater vestibular gland (female); ischioanal fossa
Anal	Sacrotuberous ligaments; intertuberous line	Anal canal; anal sphincters; pudendal nerve; internal pudendal artery and vein; inferior rectal neurovasculature; ischioanal fossa; coccyx

Table 6.3 Borders and content of the anal and urogenital triangles.

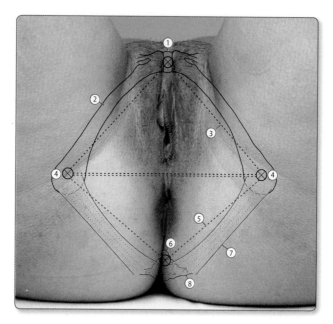

Figure 6.6 Urogenital and anal triangles of the female perineum. ① Pubic symphysis, ② ischiopubic ramus/pubic arch, ③ border of urogenital triangle (black dashed line), ④ ischial tuberosity, ⑤ border of anal triangle (red dashed line), ⑥ coccyx, ⑦ sacrotuberous ligament, ⑧ sacrum

Perineal membrane and pouches

The urogenital triangle is covered by the fibrous perineal membrane, which divides the region into deep and superficial pouches. The urogenital hiatus permits the passage of the urethra and vagina (**Figure 6.8**).

- The **deep perineal pouch** sits between the perineal membrane and the pelvic floor muscles
- The **superficial perineal pouch** sits between the perineal membrane superiorly and the perineal (Colles) fascia inferiorly

Perineal (Colles') fascia

The perineal fascia sits beneath the skin and binds to the posterior border of the perineal membrane and the fascia lata of

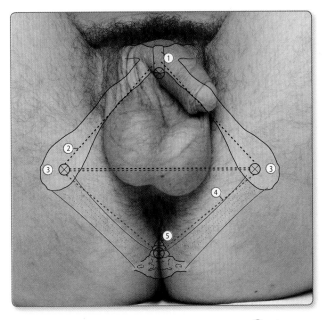

Figure 6.7 Urogenital and anal triangles of the male perineum. ① Pubic symphysis, ② border of urogenital triangle (black dashed line), ③ ischial tuberosity, ④ border of anal triangle (red dashed line), ⑤ coccyx.

the thigh. It is continuous with the dartos fascia of the scrotum and penis in the male, and with Scarpa's fascia of the abdominal wall in both sexes (**Figure 6.8**). Superficial pouch infections, Fournier's gangrene or urine leaking from a damaged penile urethra can track around the pouch (including the scrotum and penis in the male) and ascend the anterior abdominal wall.

Perineal body and pelvic floor

Perineal body This is a midline musculofibrous mass located between the vagina and anus in females and the anus and penile bulb in males (**Figures 6.8** and **6.19**). It acts as a common attachment point for levator ani, the perineal membrane and sphincter muscles and is therefore key to pelvic

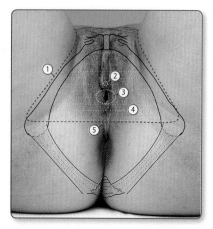

Figure 6.8 Female perineum: perineal fascia and membrane. (1) Line of attachment of perineal (Colles') fascia, (2) hiatus for urethra and external urethral orifice, (3) hiatus for vagina, (4) position of perineal membrane (grey stippling), (5) perineal body.

floor integrity and pelvic visceral support, especially in females.

The pelvic floor This is formed from a bowl-shaped sheet of voluntary muscle (levator ani and ischiococcygeus) and their fascia (**Figure 6.9**). The muscles sit deep to the perineal membrane and ischioanal fossae. The levator ani is formed from three muscles:

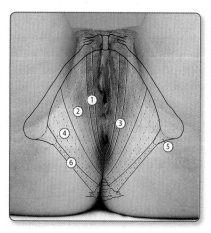

Figure 6.9 Female perineum: pelvic floor muscles. (1) Puborectalis, (2) pubococcygeus, (3) perineal body, (4) iliococcygeus, (5) ischial spine, (6) ischiococcygeus (coccygeus). **Note:** Levator ani is collectively formed by muscles 1, 2 and 4.

- Puborectalis (assists in fecal continence by maintaining the anorectal angle)
- Pubococcygeus
- Iliococcygeus

Weakening of the perineal body or pelvic floor integrity can lead to incontinence or visceral prolapse/protrusion (e.g. cystocele or rectocele). During childbirth an episiotomy can protect the perineal body from tearing. A cut is made either in the midline or posterolaterally to avoid the anal sphincter and canal.

Ischioanal fossa

The ischioanal fossae are wedge-shaped, fat-filled spaces located either side of the anal canal below the pelvic floor (**Figure 6.10**). Both extend from the sacrotuberous ligament to the pubic bone via the deep perineal pouch. The fossae are a common site for infection and cyst and fistula formation. Infection can track across the midline via a postanal communication deep to the anococcygeal ligament/body.

Anal canal

The anal canal sits in the anal triangle between the perineal and anococcygeal bodies (**Figure 6.11**). It is surrounded by a dense rings of muscle forming the internal and external anal sphincters. Sphincter tone can be assessed via digital rectal examination in suspected cauda equina syndrome. The canal is short (~ 4 cm) and passes anterosuperiorly through the pelvic floor to the anorectal junction. It permits digital rectal examination of low lying pelvic viscera.

Pectinate line

The pectinate line encircles the anal canal and marks the division between its visceral and somatic parts. The pigmented skin inferior to the pectinate line, the anoderm, is somatically innervated and therefore highly sensitive to pain.

Portocaval anastomoses and haemorrhoids

The anal canal is a point of junction between portal and systemic veins (portocaval/portosystemic anastomoses) at the internal submucosal rectal venous plexi. Congestion and dilatation of

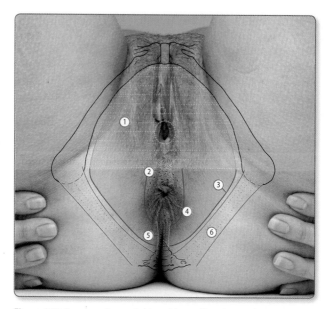

Figure 6.10 Female perineum: ischioanal fossae. Note the anterior extension of the ischioanal fossae into the deep perineal pouch and the left-right communication occurring posterior to the anal canal. ① Perineal membrane (white stipple), ② perineal body, ③ margin of ischioanal fossa (purple shade represents the ischioanal fossa), ④ external anal sphincter muscle, ⑤ anococcygeal ligament/body, ⑥ sacrotuberous ligament.

the venous plexus can lead to the formation of haemorrhoids above the pectinate line, which when prolapsed through the canal are seen at the 3, 7 and 11 o'clock positions with the patient in the lithotomy position. External haemorrhoids form around the anal margin. They can be visible, painful and feel like small round balls/berries.

6.3 Female

Mons pubis and labia

Mons pubis This is a fat-filled, hair-covered region that sits over the pubic body, symphysis and superior ramus (**Figure 6.12**).

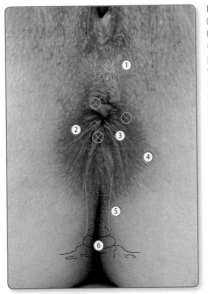

Figure 6.11 The anus. ① Perineal body, ② region of anoderm (pigmented), ③ site of pectinate line, ④ anal verge, ⑤ anococcygeal ligament/body, ⑥ coccyx, ⊗ position of appearance of prolapsed internal haemorrhoids.

Regional pain can originate from the pubic symphysis, especially during pregnancy, and regional swelling can indicate inguinal hernia.

Labia majora These flank the midline pudendal cleft, which contains the labia minora and vaginal vestibule. They contain connective tissue, subcutaneous smooth muscle and the round uterine ligament. The labia join anteriorly and posteriorly at commissures. Lipomas and varicosities of the round ligament can present as labial swelling or irreducible inguinal hernias.

Labia minora These are folds of hairless skin, the size and shape of which vary (**Figure 6.13**). They join posterior to the vaginal orifice to form the fourchette and anteriorly to form the prepuce (hood/foreskin) and frenulum of the clitoris. The fourchette can be damaged during childbirth or sex.

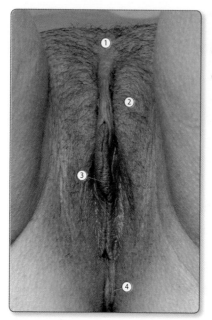

Figure 6.12 Female external genitalia: labia. ① Mons pubis, ② labia majora, ③ labia minora in pudendal cleft, ④ perineal body.

Vaginal vestibule

This sits between the labia minora. It contains the vaginal and urethral openings, the bulb of the vestibule and the greater vestibular glands (**Figures 6.13** and **6.14**).

Clitoris

The left and right crura of the clitoris attach to the inferior pubic rami and are covered superficially by the ischiocavernosus muscle. The crura leave their bony attachment as they near the pubic symphysis and join in the midline to form the clitoral body. The glans of the clitoris is covered by the prepuce (foreskin).

Bulb of the vestibule

The bulbs of the vestibule are erectile tissue located either side of the vaginal opening. They attach to the perineal membrane in the superficial pouch and are covered by the bulbospongiosus muscle.

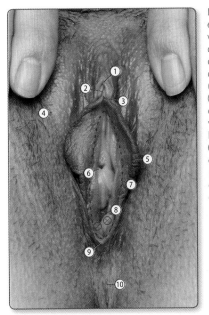

Figure 6.13 Female external genitalia: vaginal vestibule. (1) Prepuce of clitoris, (2) glans of clitoris, (3) frenulum of clitoris, (4) labia majora (opened), (5) labia minora, (6) external urethral orifice, (7) margin of vaginal vestibule (blue line), (8) vaginal orifice, (9) posterior commissure of labia/fourchette, (10) perineal body, (X) opening of greater vestibular gland ducts.

Greater vestibular gland

The greater vestibular glands are located in the superficial perineal pouch posterolateral to the vaginal opening. Their ducts open at the 5 and 7 o'clock positions relative to the vagina and they secrete mucous during sexual excitation. They can become infected and inflamed, or can develop cysts (Bartholin gland cyst) that present as a mass within the labia.

Urethra

The female urethra is ~ 4 cm long and passes anteroinferiorly through the pelvic floor, parallel to the anterior vaginal wall. It opens into the vaginal vestibule at the urethral meatus between the clitoris and vagina. Female catheterisation is relatively simple due to the urethra being short, straight and distensible. The greatest resistance to catheterisation is provided by the external urethral sphincter.

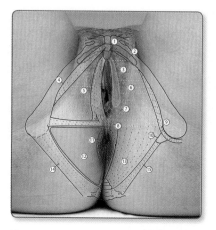

Figure 6.14 Female external genitalia: clitoris, muscles and greater vestibular glands. (Right side shows superficial structures; left shows deeper structures). ① Glans of clitoris, ② crus of clitoris, ③ bulb of vestibule, ④ ischiocavernosus muscle covering crus of clitoris, ⑤ bulbospongiosus muscle covering bulb of vestibule, ⑥ perineal membrane (white stipple), ⑦ greater vestibular gland and ducts, ⑧ perineal body, ⑨ obturator internus, ⑩ ischial spine, ⑪ external anal sphincter, ⑫ region of ischioanal fossa sat superficial to pelvic floor muscle (purple), ⑬ muscle of pelvic floor sat deep to ischioanal fat and perineal membrane, ⑭ sacrotuberous ligament, ⑮ sacrospinous ligament overlying coccygeus muscle.

Pelvic organs
Female: vagina and uterus

The vagina This is a 7–10 cm long muscular canal that passes posterosuperiorly from its opening. It is formed by posterior and anterior walls of tissue (**Figure 6.15**). Digital or speculum examination reveals the uterine cervix entering its anterior wall.

Uterus In the adult this normally lies over the superior surface of the bladder with its funducs directed towards the pubic bone. Knowledge of this arrangement enables uterine size and position to assessed via bimanual palpation. The examiner's fingers are placed against the cervix whilst the other hand applies posteroinferior pressure above the pubis. A normally positioned

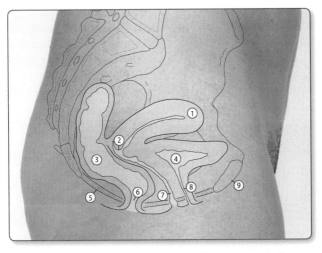

Figure 6.15 Organs of female pelvis: lateral view. ① Fundus of uterus, ② cervix of uterus, ③ rectum, ④ bladder, ⑤ levator ani (pelvic floor muscle), ⑥ anal canal (note change of angle at ano-rectal junction), ⑦ vaginal canal, ⑧ urethra, ⑨ pubic symphysis.

uterus (anteverted and anteflexed) can be palpated between the fingers.

Male and female: bladder

The size and position of the bladder varies. It normally sits posterior to the pubic symphysis and body, but expands superior to this level when full or distended (**Figure 6.16**). It can therefore be catheterised via a suprapubic approach through the midline linea alba.

6.4 Male

Penis

The penis consists of an attached part (the root) and a pendulous part (the body and glans). The penile body is covered in thin mobile skin which distally forms the retractable prepuce (foreskin) covering of the glans (**Figure 6.17**). In the ventral midline

Clinical insight

Phimosis is an inability to retract the foreskin, and paraphimosis an inability to pull a retracted foreskin back over the glans.

the foreskin connects to the glans via the frenulum. The frenulum can get damaged or torn resulting in profuse bleeding.

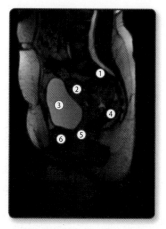

Figure 6.16 Sagittal MRI of the female pelvis. (1) Sacrum, (2) uterus, (3) bladder (full), (4) rectum, (5) vagina, (6) pubic symphysis.

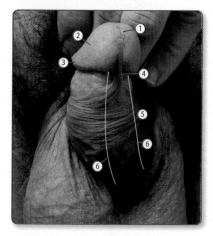

Figure 6.17 Male external genitalia: ventral penis. (1) External urethral orifice/meatus, (2) glans penis, (3) corona, (4) frenulum, (5) foreskin/prepuce (retracted), (6) lateral margins of the corpus spongiosum housing the penile urethra.

Corpus cavernosum and spongiosum

Corpus cavernosum This forms the penile crura (**Figures 6.18** and **6.19**). They attach to the ischiopubic rami and are covered superficially by ischiocavernosus, a muscle that helps maintain erection. The crura leave their bony attachment near to the pubic symphysis and meet to form the penile body. Some patient groups can develop a persistent (> 4 hours) and painful erection (priapism). Following the failure of non-invasive treatment a wide bore cannula can be inserted into the corpus cavernosum and the blood is drained.

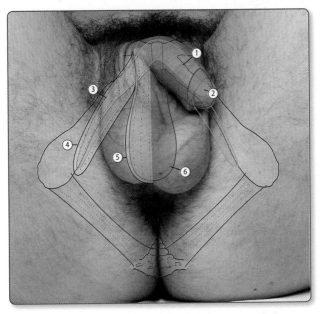

Figure 6.18 Male perineum: corpus cavernosum and corpus spongiosum (right side shows superficial structures; left side shows muscles removed). ① Corpus cavernosum in body of penis, ② glans of penis, ③ crus of penis (corpus cavernosum), ④ ischiocavernosus muscle covering the corpus cavernosum, ⑤ bulbospongiosus muscle covering the corpus spongiosum, ⑥ bulb of penis (corpus spongiosum).

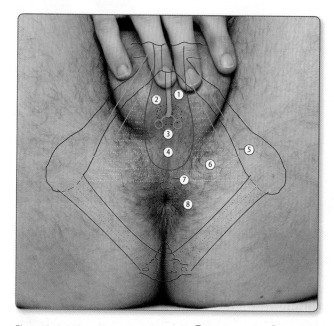

Figure 6.19 Male perineum: root of the penis. ① Spongy urethra, ② external urethral sphincter (in deep perineal pouch), ③ bulbourethral/Cowper's gland (in deep perineal pouch) with ducts draining to the urethra, ④ bulb of penis (corpus spongiosum), ⑤ crus of penis (corpus cavernosum), ⑥ perineal membrane (white stipple), ⑦ perineal body, ⑧ external anal sphincter.

Corpus spongiosum This forms the penile bulb, glans and corona and the ventral tissue mass containing the urethra. The bulb is attached to the inferior surface of the perineal membrane and is covered by bulbospongiosus, which brings about ejaculation via rhythmic urethral compression.

Urethra

The membranous urethra enters the penile bulb and bends anteriorly by ~ 90° to continue as the spongy penile urethra along the ventral penis (**Figure 6.19**). This change of angle can prove problematic during catheterisation. The urethra opens onto the glans at the external urethral meatus. Male catheterisation is more difficult than female due to the urethra changing angle at the bulb, having a non-distensible membranous part and being surrounded by the prostate.

Bulbourethral (Cowper) gland

The bulbourethral glands sit in the deep perineal pouch within the external urethral sphincter muscle at the 5 and 7 o'clock positions relative to the urethra (**Figure 6.19**). They secrete mucous into the urethra during sexual excitation. Due to their location, stones, infection or cysts within the gland can present as a perineal mass and can cause pain that is exacerbated by defecation or digital rectal examination.

Scrotum and testicles

Scrotum This is a pouch of hair-covered skin that contains, and permits the examination of, the testicles and spermatic cord. The scrotal wall appears wrinkled due to contraction of the subcutaneous dartos muscle within its wall.

Testicles These sit in the scrotum suspended by the spermatic cord (**Figure 6.20**). Their size and position vary with the left normally hanging lower than the right. The testicles are covered by the same layers as the spermatic cord therefore indirect inguinal hernias are able to track down to the testicle level (**Table 6.4**).

Palpation

Knowledge of the normal location and feel of testicular structures is essential for correct examination. The anterior, medial and lateral testicular walls should feel firm and smooth. The epididymal head can be felt over the posterosuperior testicle and the epididymal body and tail over the posterior testicle. The tail connects to the ductus deferens inferiorly, where it can be felt as a firm cord. The ductus then passes superiorly along the medial testicle to join the spermatic cord.

Spermatic cord

The spermatic cord can be palpated passing from the superficial inguinal ring (superolateral to the pubic tubercle) toward the

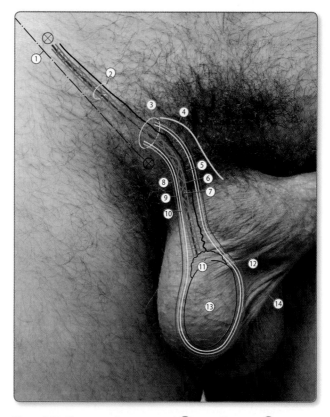

Figure 6.20 The testis and spermatic cord. ① Inguinal ligament, ②
Spermatic cord in the inguinal canal, ③ spermatic cord emerging from
superficial inguinal ring, ④ ilioinguinal nerve, ⑤ ductus deferens, ⑥
pampiniform plexus, ⑦ testicular artery, ⑧ external spermatic fascia (external
oblique), ⑨ cremasteric fascia (internal oblique), ⑩ internal spermatic fascia
(transversalis fascia), ⑪ epididymis (head), ⑫ skin of scrotum, ⑬ testicle
(surrounded by the tunica vaginalis), ⑭ midline scrotal raphe, Ⓧ position of
deep inguinal ring, Ⓧ pubic tubercle.

superior pole of the testicle. The cord contents are discussed
in **Chapter 3**. The ductus deferens can be identified in the cord

Covering	Description
External spermatic fascia	Continuation of external oblique aponeurosis and covering fascia
Cremasteric fascia	Continuation of internal oblique fascia and muscle fibres from internal oblique
Internal spermatic fascia	Continuation of transversalis fascia
Tunica vaginalis	Double layered serous membrane that assists with free testicular movement Accumulation of fluid within the tunica forms a hydrocele

Table 6.4 Coverings of the testicle.

via the upper scrotal wall and can be cut in this region during male sterilisation/vasectomy. Note, the ilioinguinal nerve runs alongside the cord and should be identified and avoided during vasectomy as damage can lead to sensory loss or pain.

Swellings
Multiple swellings can occur in or around the testicle and scrotum.
- A **varicocele** is a swelling of the pampiniform plexus
- A **spermatocele** is a swelling of the epididymis
- A **hydrocele** is an accumulation of serous fluid in the tunica vaginalis around the testicle. Examiners can normally get their fingers above a hydrocele and it transilluminates with a red glow

6.5 Perineal neurovasculature

Pudendal nerve and internal pudendal artery
The pudendal nerve (S2–4) and internal pudendal artery form the main neurovascular supply to the perineum (**Figure 6.21**). They enter the region by looping around the sacrospinous ligament and travel anteriorly along the lateral wall of the ischioanal fossa within the fascia-bound pudendal (Alcock) canal toward the penile/clitoral glans. They give off common branches that travel medially to supply perineal structures.

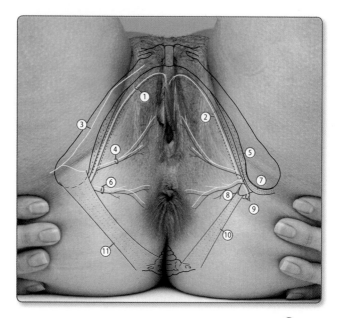

Figure 6.21 Female perineum: neurovasculature and pudendal canal. ① Dorsal nerve and artery of clitoris, ② border of pudendal canal (grey hatched line), ③ Perineal sensory branch of the posterior cutaneous nerve of the thigh, ④ perineal nerve and artery, ⑤ obturator internus, ⑥ inferior rectal nerve and artery, ⑦ tendon of obturator internus, ⑧ ischial spine, ⑨ pudendal nerve and internal pudendal artery, ⑩ sacrospinous ligament (sacrotuberous ligament removed), ⑪ sacrotuberous ligament overlying sacrospinous ligament.

- The **inferior rectal branches** arise at the entrance to the pudendal canal and travel inferomedially to supply the external anal sphincter and anal triangle skin
- The **perineal branches** arise in the distal pudendal canal. They pass to both perineal pouches and supply voluntary muscles, erectile tissue, glands, external urethral sphincter and skin of the vaginal vestibule/labia/scrotum
- The **dorsal penile/clitoral branches** pass anteriorly through the deep perineal pouch then along either side the dorsum of the penis or clitoris to the glans (**Figure 6.22**)

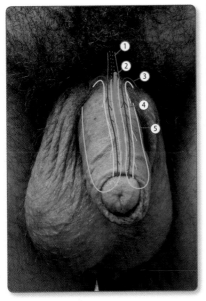

Figure 6.22 Male external genitalia: neurovasculature of the dorsal penis. ① Suspensory ligament of the penis, ② deep dorsal vein of penis, ③ dorsal artery of penis, ④ dorsal nerve of penis, ⑤ margin of corpus cavernosum.

Regional anaesthesia

- **Penile anaesthesia** for procedures such as circumcision or frenular repair can be achieved via injection either side of the suspensory ligament that attaches the penis to the pubic symphysis (**Figure 6.22**). The dorsal penile nerves sit either side of both the ligament and the prominent deep dorsal penile vein
- **Pudendal nerve anaesthesia** can be performed for perineal procedures or during childbirth. The nerve is anesthetised as it loops around the sacrospinous ligament close to the ischial spine. The spine can be palpated via the vagina and the needle inserted transvaginally

Posterior cutaneous nerve of the thigh

The perineal branch of the posterior cutaneous nerve of the thigh travels anteromedially from ~ 4 cm inferior to the ischial

Clinical insight

Testicular examination of young males with cold hands can reproduce the appearance of testicular maldescent due to retraction by the cremasteric fascia/ muscle.

tuberosity toward the pubic symphysis, along the lateral side of the ischiopubic ramus. It innervates perineal skin and therefore may need to be blocked to achieve full perineal anaesthesia. Compression of the nerve is a possible cause of perineal pain.

Dermatomes

Skin covering the pelvic girdle and perineum is innervated by spinal nerves T12–L3 and S2-5 (**Figure 1.37**). Key dermatomes include:

- **T12**: iliac crest and upper inguinal ligament
- **L1**: lower inguinal ligament anterior scrotum/labia, and proximal penis
- **S2–3**: glans and body of the penis and clitoris

The vertebral column and back

Anatomically, the back is formed by the posterior regions of the thorax and abdomen. For simplicity, in this chapter, the posterior neck and sacrum will be included as part of the back since they share common anatomy. The back is formed from multiple layers of structures including:

- The vertebral column, meninges and spinal cord
- The posterior thoracic wall (ribs and intercostal muscles)
- The scapula and superficial muscles acting on the pectoral girdle
- The deep intrinsic muscles acting on the vertebral column

Function

The vertebral column forms the midline structure of the back to which the head, limbs, thoracic cage and abdominal wall are attached. The column is a dynamic weight-bearing structure able to absorb shock and transmit forces between the upper body and the lower limbs. The column also conveys and protects the spinal cord and nerves in their meningeal coverings. The dynamic stress-bearing nature of the back and vertebral column means that it is a common site of pain via mechanical or neural injury.

7.1 Vertebral column

The vertebral column is normally formed of 33 vertebrae and associated ligaments, intervertebral discs and facet (zygapophyseal) joints. The column is divided into five regions (**Table 7.1** and **Figure 7.1**).

Vertebrae

The neural arch of a vertebra is formed by the spinous process, lamina, transverse process and pedicles. Several features of the arch can be palpated via the skin and serve as useful landmarks for examination and procedures such as spinal nerve block and epidural anaesthesia.

Region	Number of vertebrae	Vertebral nomenclature
Cervical	7	C1–C7
Thoracic	12	T1–T12
Lumbar	5	L1–L5
Sacral	5 (fused)	S1–S5
Coccygeal	4 (variable)	Co1–Co4

Table 7.1 Vertebral column regions and nomenclature.

Identification of spinous processes

The tips of the spinous processes are palpable within the midline groove/furrow of the back, especially during vertebral column flexion. In the upper cervical region the processes overlie their own vertebral body. Travelling inferiorly the processes get longer and angled more posteroinferiorly such that they overlie the inferiorly located vertebral body. In the lower thoracic and lumbar regions the processes shorten and tend to overlie the lower part of their own vertebral body and the inferiorly located intervertebral disc (**Figure 7.2**). Key spinous processes can be located as shown in **Table 7.2**.

Spinous process levels

The spinous processes, or the space between them, can be used to mark the levels of underlying structures or planes and therefore help guide posterior approaches during surgery or anaesthesia (**Table 7.3** and **Figure 7.3**).

Sacral triangle and sacral hiatus

Sacral triangle This is a reliable marker of the sacral hiatus during caudal epidural anaesthesia, especially in larger patients where palpation can be difficult (**Figure 7.4**). An equilateral triangle is drawn between the poste-

Clinical insight

Coeliac plexus block for severe abdominal pain is performed from a posterior approach using the 12th rib and transverse process of L1 as landmarks.

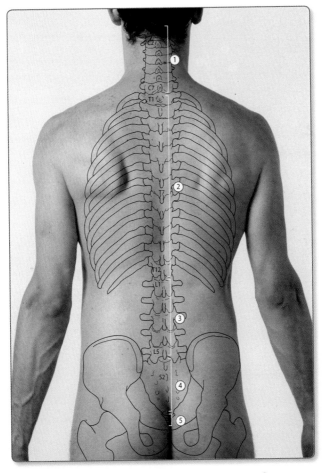

Figure 7.1 Vertebral column regions. ① Cervical region (C1–C7), ② thoracic region (T1–T12), ③ lumbar region (L1–L5), ④ sacral region (S1–S5), ⑤ coccyx (Co1–Co4).

rior superior iliac spines, the distance between which forms the baseline measurement, and the midline of the sacrum towards its apex. The sacral hiatus sits at the inferior tip of the triangle.

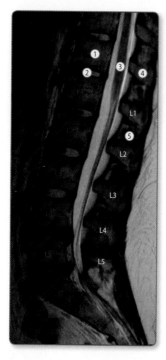

Figure 7.2 Sagittal MRI of the lumbar spine. (1) Vertebral body, (2) intervertebral disc, (3) spinal cord in vertebral canal, (4) spinous process, (5) space between spinous processes. **Note:** the lumbar spinous processes (white labels L1–L5) sit over the lower part of their own vertebral body (red labels L1–L5) and the intervertebral disc below. The space between adjacent lumbar spinous processes overlies the vertebral body of the vertebrae below.

Spinous process	Location
C2	First midline mass palpated inferior to the cranium; forms a corner of the suboccipital triangle
C7	The most prominent spinous process on the inferior neck (vertebrae prominens)
T12	At the medial end of the 12th rib when traced superomedially
L4	On the supracristal plane (highest point of iliac crest)
S2	On, or just below, the plane joining the posterior superior iliac spines
S3	Palpable at the top of the natal/gluteal cleft

Table 7.2 Location of landmark spinous processes.

Spinous process (spaces)	Vertebral level	Feature/plane
C7	C7–T1	Superior limit of lung apex in posterior triangle of neck
T3	Upper T4	Medial end of scapula spine; superior extent of oblique lung fissure
T4	Upper T5	Tracheal bifurcation (may hear bronchial breath sounds to right of midline at this level); immediately below the sternal plane
T7	T8	Inferior angle of scapula; triangle of auscultation; inferior vena cava crosses diaphragm
T11	Upper T12	Aorta crosses diaphragm; coeliac trunk and plexus; lower limit of costodiaphragmatic recess
T12–L1 space	L1	Transpyloric plane; superior mesenteric artery and plexus; kidney hilum
L1–L2 space	L2	Inferior limit of spinal cord (adult)
L2–L3 space	L3	Inferior pole of kidney; inferior mesenteric artery and plexus; inferior limit of infant/child spinal cord
L3–L4 space	L4	Bifurcation of aorta; lumbar puncture insertion site
L4	L4-L5 intervertebral disc	Supracristal plane; used to landmark the needle insertion site for adult lumbar puncture either above (L3–4 space) or below (L4–5 space)
S2	S2	Termination of subarachnoid space

Table 7.3 Key structures, planes and vertebrae landmarked by spinous processes or the spaces between adjacent processes.

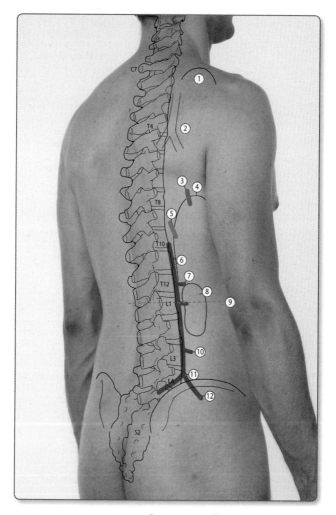

Figure 7.3 Spinous process levels. ① Apex of lung, ② tracheal bifurcation, ③ inferior vena cava pierces diaphragm at T8, ④ diaphragm (highest point), ⑤ oesophagus pierces diaphragm at T10, ⑥ aorta pierces diaphragm at T12, ⑦ coeliac trunk, ⑧ kidney, ⑨ transpyloric plane (dashed green line), hilum of kidney and superior mesenteric artery, ⑩ inferior mesenteric artery, ⑪ aortic bifurcation, ⑫ common iliac artery.

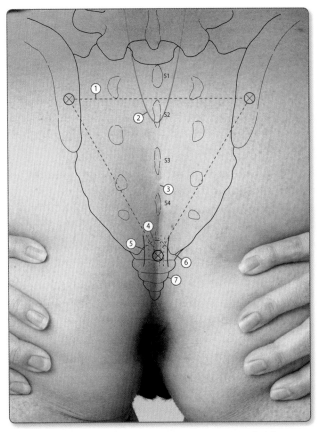

Figure 7.4 Sacral triangle and hiatus within the intergluteal (natal) cleft. ① Borders of sacral triangle (red line), ② lower limit of subarachnoid space, ③ sacrum, ④ sacral hiatus, ⑤ sacrococcygeal ligament, ⑥ sacral cornua, ⑦ coccyx, ⊗ posterior superior iliac spine, ⊗ inferior tip/apex of sacral triangle.

Sacral hiatus This is the inferior opening of the vertebral canal. It is located near the sacral apex within the intergluteal cleft. The hiatus sits inferior to S4 spinous process and between the laterally located bony crests of the sacral cornua, which are palpable. Caudal epidural anaesthesia can be achieved via needle insertion thorough the sacral hiatus. The needle penetrates the sacrococcygeal ligament and is progressed into the epidural space noting that the subdural space ends at S2 and is therefore ~ 3.5 cm away.

Transverse processes and laminae

Laminae These are flattened plates of bone connecting the spinous and transverse processes (**Figure 7.5**). They sit under the muscle masses flanking the median furrow. The lamina can present an obstruction during lumbar puncture/epidural anaesthesia if the needle is angled incorrectly. The lamina can be removed (laminectomy) as a decompressive treatment for vertebral canal stenosis and associated nerve compression.

> ### Clinical insight
>
> Spina bifida occulta represents a failure of neural arch formation around L5–S1. Skin over the defect is covered by a small tuft of hair.

Transverse processes These mark the positions of spinal nerves and are therefore useful during procedures such as regional nerve or plexus anaesthesia (**Table 7.4** and **Figure 7.5**).

Joints

Three joints can be surface marked on the back. All can be the cause of localised pain that often refers to the region overlying the joint (**Figure 7.5**). The joints can be injected under radiographic guidance with varying outcome.

- **Costotransverse joints** (synovial) sit between a rib and its corresponding transverse processes. They are located deep to the tip of the thoracic transverse process ~ 2.5 cm lateral to the midvertebral line
- **Facet (zygapophyseal) joints** (synovial) sit between the superior and inferior articular facets of adjacent vertebrae. They are located ~ 1–2 cm lateral to the midvertebral line, between the spinous and transverse processes
- The **sacrococcygeal joint** (secondary cartilaginous) sits between the sacrum and coccyx. It can be palpated as a groove just below the inferior tip of the sacral triangle. The joint is

Transverse process	Location and structures landmarked
C1	Firm mass palpated through sternocleidomastoid inferior to the mastoid process; contains the vertebral artery
C2–C5	Pass posteroinferiorly down the lateral neck from the C1 transverse process, deep to the neck muscles ~ 2–3 cm from the skin; can be identified using horizontal planes aligned with neck viscera; used as a landmark during cervical plexus block
C6	Possesses a palpable tubercle on its anterior surface which is located lateral to the cricoid and deep to the common carotid artery; used as a landmark in stellate ganglion and brachial plexus block
Thoracic	Sit on the parasagittal plane, 2.5 cm lateral to the midvertberal line; used to landmark the position of spinal nerves during paravertebral thoracic nerve block Note: the thoracic spinous process tips mark the level of the transverse process of the vertebrae below
Lumbar	Align with a vertical plane drawn through the posterior inferior iliac spine; used to landmark the position of the lumbar spinal nerves/lumbar plexus during a psoas compartment /plexus block

Table 7.4 Location of, and structures landmarked by, the vertebral transverse processes.

used as a landmark for ganglion impar injection and can be a source of severe coccygeal pain (coccydynia)

Ligaments

Ligaments pass between the spinous processes and lamina of adjacent vertebrae (**Figures 7.6** and **7.7**).

- The **supraspinous ligament** attaches to the tips of adjacent spinous processes forming a continuous palpable midline ridge
- The **interspinous ligament** sits deep to the supraspinous ligament and attaches to adjacent spinous processes
- **Ligamentum flavum** connects the lamina of adjacent vertebrae and unites in the midline. It has elastic properties

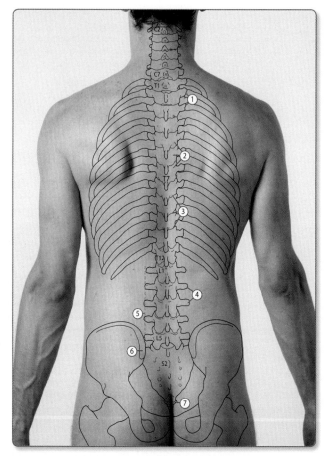

Figure 7.5 Posterior view of the vertebra and intervertebral joints.
① Costotransverse joints, ② vertebral laminae, ③ facet/zygapophyseal joints,
④ transverse processes, ⑤ vertical plane aligned with the posterior superior
iliac spine landmarks the lumbar vertebral transverse processes, ⑥ posterior
superior iliac spine, ⑦ sacrococcygeal joint.

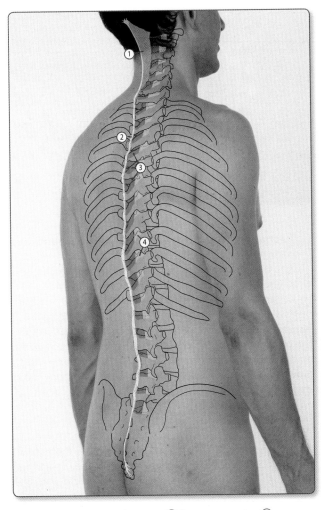

Figure 7.6 Vertebral column ligaments. ① Ligamentum nuchae, ② supra-spinous ligament (white), ③ interspinous ligament (pink), ④ ligamentum flavum (yellow).

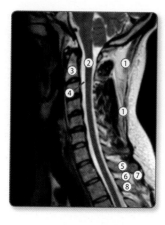

Figure 7.7 Sagittal MRI of the cervical spine. ① Ligamentum nuchae, ② spinal cord, ③ C2 vertebral body and dens, ④ cerebrospinal fluid, ⑤ T1 spinous process, ⑥ interspinous ligament, ⑦ supraspinous ligament, ⑧ T2 spinous process.

- The **ligamentum nuchae** is a large midline ligament attached to the spinous processes of the cervical vertebrae and the skull base from the inion to the foramen magnum. It is palpable in the midvertebral line during neck flexion

The supraspinous, interspinous and flaval ligaments are pierced during the midvertebral line approach used for lumbar puncture or epidural anaesthesia (**Figure 7.12**). A sudden give can be felt after passing through ligamentum flavum into the epidural space. The interspinous and nuchal ligaments also provide a relatively avascular surgical plane between erector spinae for posterior approaches to the vertebral column.

Curvatures

The vertebral column is curved in the sagittal plane (**Figure 7.8**). At birth the column is C-shaped (kyphosed) in the primary curvature. The secondary curvatures form in the cervical and lumbar regions during the early years of growth. When viewed posteriorly the thoracic and sacral regions curve posteriorly forming a convexity (kyphosis) whereas the cervical and lumbar regions curve anteriorly forming a concavity (lordosis) (**Table 7.5**).

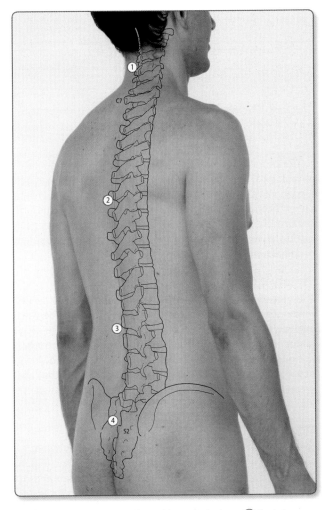

Figure 7.8 Normal curvatures of the adult vertebral column. ① Cervical lordosis, ② thoracic kyphosis, ③ lumbar lordosis, ④ sacral kyphosis.

Vertebrae	Curvature	Type
C1–T2	Cervical lordosis	Secondary
T2–T12	Thoracic kyphosis	Primary
T12–L5	Lumbar lordosis	Secondary
L5–S5	Sacral kyphosis	Primary

Table 7.5 Normal curvatures of the adult vertebral column.

Abnormal curvatures can be congenital, developmental or pathological. For example, osteoporosis can cause an exaggerated thoracic kyphosis (humpback) and pregnant or overweight patients can develop a compensatory exaggeration of the lumbar lordosis. Scoliosis is an abnormal lateral curvature, which can be due to weak back muscles, failure of vertebral development or spinal tumours.

Vertebral canal

The vertebral canal conveys the spinal cord, spinal nerves, meninges and associated vasculature (**Figure 7.9**). The canal extends from the foramen magnum superiorly to the sacral hiatus inferiorly and is covered posteriorly by the vertebral spinous processes, lamina and associated ligaments. Knowledge of the surface position, arrangement and content of the canal is essential to ensuring safe lumbar puncture and anaesthesia (epidural/spinal).

Meninges

The spinal cord and spinal nerve roots are covered by meninges within the vertebral canal and intervertebral foramen (**Figure 7.9**). The spaces and meningeal layers of the vertebral canal are organised from superficial to deep as shown in **Table 7.6**.

Spinal cord

The adult spinal cord terminates as the medullary cone at vertebral level L1–L2, proximal to the termination of the subarachnoid space at S2 (**Figure 7.9** and **7.10**). Both levels can

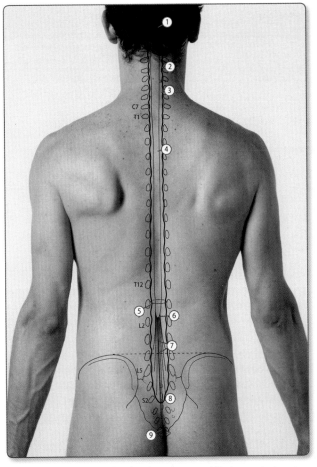

Figure 7.9 Meninges, spinal cord and spinal nerves within the vertebral canal (cutaway view). ① Foramen magnum, ② dura mater lined internally with arachnoid mater, ③ subarachnoid space filled with cerebrospinal fluid, ④ spinal cord covered in pia mater, ⑤ vertebral canal containing spinal cord and nerves within meningeal coverings, ⑥ conus medullaris (termination of spinal cord), ⑦ cauda equina, ⑧ termination of subarachnoid space, ⑨ sacral hiatus.

Space/layer	Location and/or content
Epidural space (superficial)	Fat and vein-filled space sat outside of the dura; runs the length of the vertebral column to the sacral hiatus; region for epidural injection
Dura mater	Extends from the foramen magnum to the coccygeal periosteum; continuous with cranial dura surrounding the brain
Subdural space	Potential space between the dura and arachnoid; bleeds into the space can cause acute back pain and signs of cord/cauda equina lesion
Arachnoid mater	Lines the inside of the dura
Subarachnoid space	Sits between the arachnoid and pia; extends the length of the vertebral canal to S2 (~ 35 mm proximal to the sacral hiatus), but can range in position from L5–S3; filled with cerebrospinal fluid
Pia mater (deep)	Directly covers the surface of the neural tissue (spinal cord and spinal nerves)

Table 7.6 Meningeal coverings and spaces surrounding the spinal cord.

be determined via spinous processes. During early in-utero development the spinal cord and vertebral column are similar lengths, however, both change in size differentially such that the newborn's spinal cord terminates around the L2–L3 vertebral level. This must be borne in mind when performing lumbar puncture on infants and children.

Spinal nerves
Spinal nerves arise sequentially from the spinal cord from C1 superiorly to S5, or Co0 (coccygeal), inferiorly (**Figure 7.11**). Spinal nerves exit the vertebral canal laterally via the intervertebral foramen, the surface position of which can be approximated during spinal nerve block using the vertebral transverse processes. Spinal nerves exit the vertebral canal as shown in **Table 7.7**.

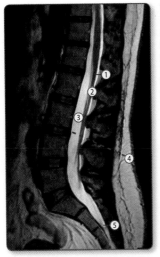

Figure 7.10 Sagittal MRI of the lumbosacral spine. ① Termination of spinal cord (conus medullaris), ② cauda equina, ③ subarachnoid space, ④ line of approach for lumbar puncture between L3–L4 spinous processes, ⑤ termination of subarachnoid space.

The spinal cord can be divided into regions with each region being named according to the spinal nerves arising from it, for example, the sacral region of the cord gives rise to the sacral spinal nerves S1–S5. As the spinal cord ends at L1–L2, the vertebral level at which the more caudal spinal nerves arise from the cord differs from their level of exit via the intervertebral foramen (**Table 7.8**). This is important when considering the consequences of a cord injury at a given level.

Cauda equina

This is a collection of spinal nerves passing through the subarachnoid space distal to the spinal cord termination at L2 (**Figures 7.10** and **7.11**). The region of subarachnoid space distal to L2 is safe for lumbar puncture. The cauda ends at S2 with the termination of the dural sac. Cauda equina compression (syndrome) in the vertebral canal can cause lower limb muscle weakness, gait ataxia, reduced anal tone, perineal anaesthesia, local back pain and pain radiating to the lower limb (radiculopathy).

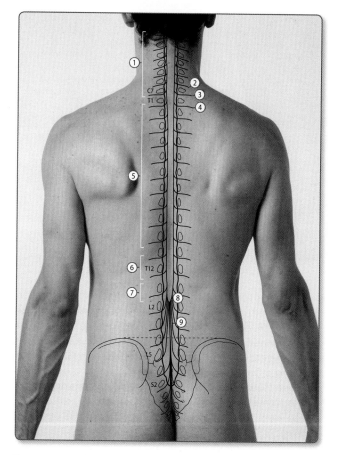

Figure 7.11 Spinal cord regions and spinal nerves (cutaway view). ① Cervical region of spinal cord, ② C7 spinal nerve, ③ C8 spinal nerve, ④ T1 spinal nerve, ⑤ thoracic region of spinal cord, ⑥ lumbar region of spinal cord, ⑦ sacral region of spinal cord, ⑧ conus medullaris (termination of spinal cord), ⑨ cauda equina.

Lumbar puncture/epidural anaesthesia

The same approach is used for both lumbar puncture and regional epidural anaesthesia. The vertebral column is flexed

Spinal nerve	Vertebral canal exit point
C1–C7	Above C1–C7, respectively
C8	Below C7
T1–S5	Below T1–S5, respectively

Table 7.7 Spinal nerve exit point from the vertebral canal relative to the vertebrae.

Spinal nerve	Spinal cord region of origin	Vertebral level of origin/ spinal cord region
C1–C8	Cervical	C1–C7
T1–T12	Thoracic	T1–T10
L1–L5	Lumbar	T11–T12
S1–S5	Sacral	L1–L2

Table 7.8 Vertebral level of spinal nerve origin from the spinal cord.

maximally and the L4 spinous process identified on the supracristal plane (**Figure 7.12**). A needle is inserted in the midline between the spinous processes of L3–L4 or L4–L5 and directed anterosuperiorly. It passes through the supraspinous, interspinous and flaval ligaments after which a 'give' or 'pop' is felt as it enters the epidural space. Epidural anaesthesia can be administered here. To sample cerebrospinal fluid the needle is advanced through the dura and arachnoid, at which point a second 'give/pop' is felt, into the subarachnoid space.

7.2 Muscles

A knowledge of the layers of muscle covering the back helps guide minimally damaging/invasive surgical approaches to the vertebral column. The extrinsic and intrinsic muscles of the back are arranged in three main layers:
- Superficial extrinsic
- Intermediate extrinsic
- Deep intrinsic (surrounded in deep fascia)

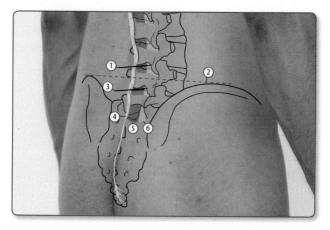

Figure 7.12 Location and route of travel for lumbar puncture. ① Approach between L3 and L4 vertebrae, ② supracristal plane marking L4 spinous process, ③ approach between L4 and L5 vertebrae, ④ supraspinous ligament, ⑤ interspinous ligament, ⑥ ligamentum flavum.

Superficial extrinsic layer

This consists of flat sheets of muscle that act on the upper limb and scapula, including the trapezius, rhomboids and latissimus dorsi (**Chapter 4**). Two clinically useful triangular regions can be identified between the borders of the muscle layers: the triangle of auscultation and the lumbar triangle (**Figure 7.13**).

The triangle of auscultation This is located medial to the inferior angle of the scapula. The lack of overlying muscle makes it a good location auscultation of the inferior lung lobe. The triangle is bordered:

- Inferiorly by latissimus dorsi
- Superolaterally by rhomboid major (for simplicity the medial scapula border is often used instead)
- Superomedially by trapezius

The lumbar (Petit's) triangle This is located superior to the iliac crest and just lateral to its highest (supracristal) point. Hernias can pass through the triangle. The triangle is bordered:

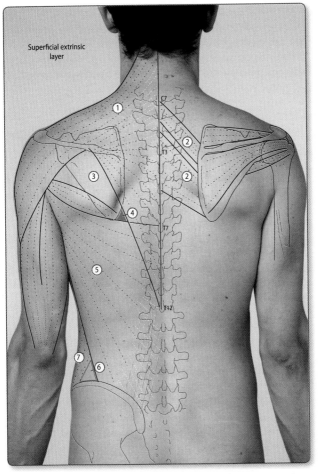

Figure 7.13 Posterior view of back muscles: superficial extrinsic layer. (1) Trapezius, (2) rhomboids (minor and major), (3) scapula, (4) triangle of auscultation, (5) latissimus dorsi, (6) lumbar (Petit's triangle), (7) External oblique.

- Inferiorly by iliac crest
- Superolaterally by external oblique
- Superomedially by latissimus dorsi

Intermediate extrinsic layer

Serratus posterior superior and serratus posterior inferior are flat sheets of muscle located deep to the rhomboids and latissimus dorsi, respectively (**Figure 7.14**). They pass from spinous processes to the ribs and have been reported to be a potential source of regional back pain.

Deep and thoracolumbar fascia

Deep fascia covers the deep intrinsic muscle layer. It attaches to the transverse and spinous vertebral processes, spinous ligaments, rib angles, sacrum and iliolumbar ligament (**Figure 7.14**). In the thoracic and lumbar regions the deep (thoracolumbar) fascia fans out inferolaterally to join the iliac crest. The fascia can be incised or cut from the spinous processes to provide access to the vertebral column.

Deep intrinsic layer

The deep intrinsic muscle layer forms the longitudinal (parasagittal) muscular prominences either side of the median furrow (**Table 7.9** and **Figures 7.14–7.16**).

Erector spinae (intermediate part)

The erector spinae group forms the majority of the prominent paravertebral muscle mass. Inferiorly it has a distinct palpable lateral border, that is used as a landmark for kidney examination and surgical incision. It is formed from three columns of muscle, several parts of which arise inferiorly from the large erector aponeurosis (**Table 7.10** and **Figure 7.15**). Each of the three columns of the erector spinae group can be further subdivided depending upon their attachments or the region they span (**Table 7.11**).

Suboccipital triangle

This is located deep to splenius capitis and semispinalis on the posterior neck (**Figure 7.17**). It is bordered:

- Superomedially by rectus capitis posterior major
- Superolaterally by obliquus capitis superior

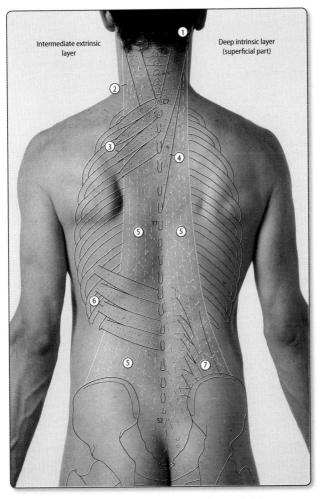

Figure 7.14 Posterior view of back muscles: intermediate extrinsic layer and deep intrinsic layer (superficial part). ① Splenius capitis, ② deep neck fascia, ③ serratus posterior superior, ④ splenius cervicis, ⑤ thoracolumbar fascia, ⑥ serratus posterior inferior, ⑦ quadratus lumborum muscle (deep thoracolumbar fascia and deep back muscles).

Part/layer	Muscles	Location
Superficial (**Figure 7.14**)	Splenius capitis; splenius cervicis	Pass superolaterally around the posterior neck from the cervicothoracic spinous processes to the mastoid, superior nuchal line and C1–C3; forms the wide 'bull-neck' appearance of muscular individuals
Intermediate (**Figure 7.15**)	Erector spinae group	Prominent vertical bands of muscle running the length of the vertebral column located either side of median furrow
Deep (**Figure 7.16**)	Semispinales; rotatores; multifidus	Sit between the spinous and transverse vertebral processes; semispinales capitis forms the palpable vertical muscular band either side of the midline posterior neck

Table 7.9 Deep intrinsic layers of back muscle divided into three layers/parts.

Column	Muscle group	Location
Medial	Spinalis	Adjacent to the spinous processes of the cervical and thoracic vertebrae
Intermediate	Longissimus	Between the erector aponeurosis, transverse processes, medial part of the ribs to their angles, and the mastoid process
Lateral	Iliocostalis	Between the erector aponeurosis, rib angles and cervical vertebrae

Table 7.10 Locations of the three muscle columns of erector spinae.

- Inferiorly by obliquus capitis inferior

The borders of the triangle can be mapped out between three palpable bony prominences; the C2 spinous process, the C1 transverse process (inferior to the mastoid) and the lateral part

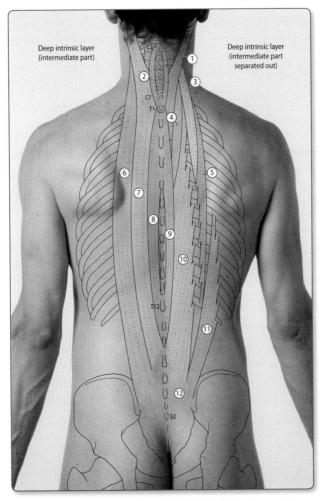

Figure 7.15 Posterior view of back muscles: deep intrinsic layer (intermediate part). ① Longissimus capitis, ② spinales cervicis, ③ iliocostalis cervicis, ④ longissimus cervicis, ⑤ iliocostalis thoracis, ⑥ lateral column (iliocostalis muscle), ⑦ intermediate column (longissimus muscle), ⑧ medial column (spinalis muscle), ⑨ spinales thoracis, ⑩ longissimus thoracis, ⑪ iliocostalis lumborum, ⑫ erector spinae aponeurosis. Note: collectively the medial, intermediate and lateral muscle columns form erector spinae.

Spinalis	Longissimus	Iliocostalis
Capitis*	Capitis	Cervicis
Cervicis*	Cervicis	Thoracis
Thoracis	Thoracis	Lumborum
*Often poorly defined/absent.		

Table 7.11 Subdivisions of the erector spinae muscle group.

of the superior nuchal line. The triangle is a useful marker for the position of key structures (**Figure 7.18**), including:

- The posterior arch of C1
- The vertebral artery sitting superior to C1
- The suboccipital nerve (C1 dorsal ramus)
- The posterior atlanto-occipital membrane

Clinical insight

Compression of the C2 or C3 dorsal ramus can cause headache/occipital neuralgia, which is relieved by local block or surgical decompression.

The triangle is crossed by the dorsal ramus of C2 (greater occipital nerve) which emerges from below obliquus capitis inferior ~ 1–2 cm lateral to the C2 spinous process, then travels superomedially onto the occipital bone. The dorsal ramus of C3 sits medially. Prolonged compression of the C2 or C3 dorsal ramus during posterior neck surgery can cause postoperative pain.

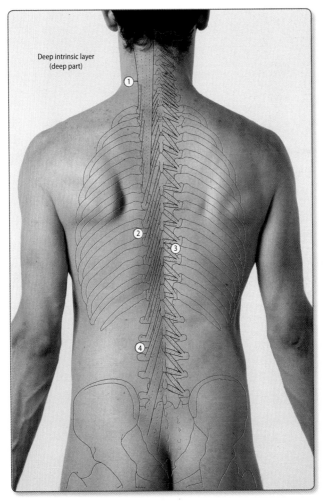

Figure 7.16 Posterior view of back muscles: deep intrinsic layer (deep part).
① Semispinales capitis, ② semispinales thoracis, ③ rotatores, ④ multifidus.

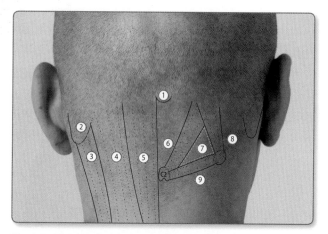

Figure 7.17 Intermediate and deep muscles of the posterior neck and the suboccipital triangle. ① External occipital protruberance (inion), ② mastoid process, ③ longissimus capitis, ④ splenius capitis, ⑤ semispinalis capitis, ⑥ rectus capitis posterior major, ⑦ suboccipital triangle (green dashed border), ⑧ obliquus capitis superior, ⑨ obliquus capitis inferior.

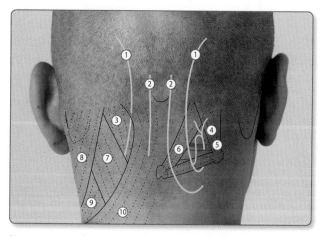

Figure 7.18 Superficial muscles of the posterior neck and neurovasculature of the suboccipital triangle. ① Greater occipital nerve (dorsal ramus of C2), ② dorsal ramus of C3, ③ semispinalis capitis, ④ suboccipital nerve (dorsal ramus of C1), ⑤ vertebral artery, ⑥ posterior arch of C1 (atlas), ⑦ splenius capitis, ⑧ sternocleidomastoid, ⑨ levator scapulae, ⑩ trapezius.

chapter 8

Head and neck

Head

The head comprises the cranium and associated tissues. It contains the brain, brainstem, cerebellum and organs of special sense, speech, feeding and breathing. The cranium is formed from a set of irregular bones united mostly via fibrous suture joints. It consists of two main parts (**Figure 8.1**):

- The **neurocranium** (**calvaria** and **skull base**), which houses the brain and associated neural tissues
- The **viscerocranium** (**facial skeleton**), which includes the nasal cavity, orbits, oral cavity, palate, teeth and mandible

Many of the outer-facing surfaces, features and joints of the skull bones are palpable through the skin and subcutaneous tissue of the scalp and face. Several bony features serve as landmarks for underlying structures, foramen and muscle attachments.

Neck

The neck connects the head and associated viscera with the trunk and upper limbs. For descriptive purposes the neck is bordered (**Figure 8.2**):

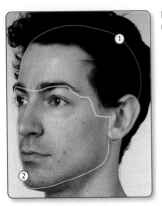

Figure 8.1 The cranium.
(1) Neurocranium, (2) viscerocranium.

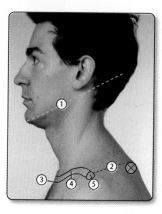

Figure 8.2 Anatomical margins of the neck. ① Pericraniocervical line, ② acromion (C7 vertebral body line), ③ sternal notch of manubrium, ④ clavicle, ⑤ acromion, Ⓧ C7 spinous process.

- **Superiorly** by the pericraniocervical line, which passes from the chin, around the inferior border of the mandible and base of the skull to the external occipital protuberance
- **Inferiorly** by the superior border of the manubrium, clavicle and acromion and a line passing from the acromion to the C7 vertebral body

The neck is continuous with the superior mediastinum of the thorax at the plane of the thoracic inlet, which crosses the manubrium, first rib and body of vertebra T1.

Vertebral levels

Several head and neck features serve as markers for regional vertebrae, which can be observed on radiographs (**Figure 8.3**).

- **C2** Mandibular angle
- **C3** Hyoid body
- **C4** Thyrohyoid membrane/carotid bifurcation
- **C5** Laryngeal prominence and vocal folds
- **C6** Cricoid cartilage/tracheal origin

8.1 Bones and bony landmarks

Frontal bone

The frontal bone forms the forehead, supraorbital margin and roof of the orbit (**Figure 8.4**). It joins the parietal bones at the

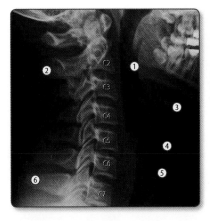

Figure 8.3 Lateral radiograph of the cervical spine. (1) Angle of mandible, (2) C2 spinous process, (3) hyoid bone, (4) laryngeal prominence, (5) cricoid cartilage, (6) C7 spinous process.

coronal suture, which runs along a line joining the midpoints of the zygomatic arches (**Figure 8.5** and **8.6**). The glabella of the frontal bone forms the rounded midline prominence above the nose. The superciliary arches are raised prominences located superomedial to the orbit. Palpation around the superomedial border of the orbit reveals a supraorbital foramen, felt as an indentation/notch.

> ## Clinical insight
>
> Repeated tapping of the glabella elicits a blink reflex that should stop. Parkinson disease causes continued blinking (Myerson sign).

Nasal bones

The paired nasal bones form the bridge of the nose and inferior part of the midline forehead. They join the frontal bone at the nasion, a midline depression below the glabella. The nasion marks the start of the superior sagittal sinus.

Maxilla

The maxilla forms the central part of the face (**Figure 8.4**). It consists of several parts:

- The **body** is located lateral to the nose and inferior to the medial orbit

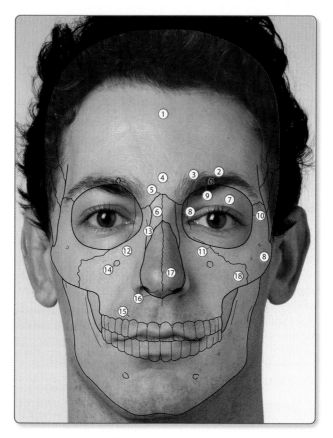

Figure 8.4 Anterior skull. ① Frontal bone, ② supraorbital foramen, ③ superciliary arch, ④ glabella, ⑤ nasion, ⑥ nasal bone, ⑦ orbit, ⑧ medial orbital margin, ⑨ superior orbital margin, ⑩ lateral orbital margin, ⑪ inferior orbital margin, ⑫ maxilla (body), ⑬ frontal process of maxilla, ⑭ infraorbital foramen, ⑮ alveolar process of maxilla, ⑯ nasal notch of maxilla, ⑰ nasal septum (cartilaginous part), ⑱ zygomatic process of maxilla.

- The **frontal process** runs superomedially between the nose and orbit. It forms the medial margin of the orbit and the superolateral part of the nose

- The **palatine processes** of the left and right maxilla join to form the anterior two thirds of the hard palate in the roof of the oral cavity (**Figure 8.25**)
- The **alveolar processes** project inferiorly into the oral cavity and hold the maxillary teeth

Mandible

The mandible forms the mobile lower part of the jaw (**Figure 8.5**). It consists of several parts, most of which are palpable and/or visible:

- The **body** runs from the midline of the chin (mental protuberance) to the ramus

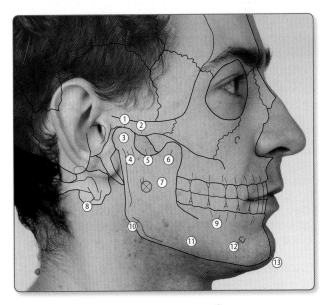

Figure 8.5 Mandible and temporomandibular joint. ① Temporomandibular joint, ② articular tubercle of temporal bone, ③ head of mandible, ④ neck of mandible, ⑤ mandibular notch, ⑥ coronoid process, ⑦ mandibular ramus, ⑧ transverse process of C1 (atlas), ⑨ alveolar process, ⑩ angle of mandible, ⑪ body of mandible, ⑫ mental foramen, ⑬ mental protuberance, Ⓧ surface position of mandibular foramen (on deep surface of ramus).

- The **ramus** is the vertical section of bone. Its posterior border is palpable up to the mandibular neck on top of which is the articular head. The maxillary artery sits deep to the upper ramus/neck
- The **angle** sits between the body and ramus. It marks vertebral level C2 and the posterior limit of the greater horn of the hyoid bone
- The **alveolar process** projects superiorly and holds the mandibular teeth
- The **mandibular notch** sits between the coronoid process and the neck/head, anteroinferior to the temporal articular tubercle
- The **coronoid process** is palpable immediately lateral to the 3rd maxillary molar tooth, via the oral vestibule

Clinical insight

The maxillary (CN Vb) or mandibular nerve (CN Vc) can be anaesthetised via the mandibular notch using either an anteriorly or posteriorly angled needle, respectively.

Temporomandibular joint

The temporomandibular joint sits between the mandibular head and the mandibular fossa and articular tubercle of the temporal bone (**Figure 8.5**). The joint line and articular tubercle are palpable anterior to the tragus and inferior to the zygomatic arch. On palpation, the mandibular head can be felt moving anteriorly across a finger during mouth opening and closing. When dislocated the mandibular head moves anterior and superior to the articular tubercle, thus locking the mouth open. Relocation requires navigation under the tubercle.

C1 vertebra

The transverse process of C1 can be palpated as a firm mass deep to sternocleidomastoid, approximately 1 cm posteroinferior to the apex of the mastoid process. It marks the position of the vertebral artery and the lower-lateral point of the suboccipital triangle of the posterior neck.

Zygomatic bone

This bone forms the prominent anterolateral part of the cheek region (**Figure 8.6**). The frontal process passes superiorly to form the lateral orbital margin. The temporal process passes posteriorly to form the anterior part of the zygomatic arch.

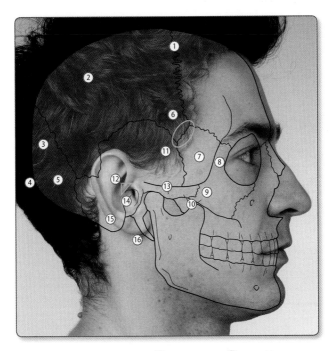

Figure 8.6 Lateral view of the skull. ① Coronal suture, ② parietal bone, ③ Occipital bone, ④ external occipital protuberance (inion), ⑤ position of superior nuchal line, ⑥ pterion (orange), ⑦ greater wing of sphenoid, ⑧ frontal process of zygoma, ⑨ temporal process of zygoma, ⑩ zygomatic arch, ⑪ squamous part of temporal bone, ⑫ suprameatal triangle (blue), ⑬ zygomatic process of temporal bone, ⑭ external acoustic meatus, ⑮ mastoid process of temporal bone, ⑯ styloid process.

Pterion

The pterion is the junction between the parietal, frontal, temporal and sphenoid bones (**Figure 8.6**). It sits 4 cm superior to the midpoint of the zygomatic arch on the lateral skull. The middle meningeal artery passes deeply, and can be lacerated via pterion region fracture resulting in an extradural hematoma. Following the injury patients may have a lucid interval of several hours duration prior to symptom onset.

Parietal bone

The paired parietal bones form the lateral sides of the dome of the calvarium, the convex shape of which is easily palpable posterior to the frontal bone (**Figure 8.6**). They unite at the midline sagittal suture (**Figure 8.9**) and join the frontal bone anteriorly at the coronal suture, the occipital bone posteriorly and the temporal and sphenoid bones inferolaterally.

Temporal bone

The temporal bone is located on the lateral cranium (**Figures 8.6** and **8.7**). It contains the ear and vestibular systems and forms part of the skull base/floor. Various pathologies can affect the bone. Fractures can cause bleeding from the ear and middle

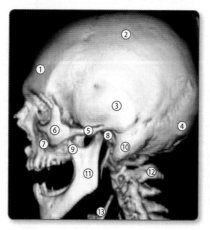

Figure 8.7 3D rendered CT image of lateral skull and neck. (**1**) Frontal bone, (**2**) parietal bone, (**3**) temporal bone (squamous part), (**4**) occipital bone, (**5**) zygomatic arch, (**6**) zygoma, (**7**) maxilla, (**8**) external acoustic meatus, (**9**) coronoid process of mandible, (**10**) mastoid process, (**11**) ramus of mandible, (**12**) C2 spinous process, (**13**) hyoid bone.

ear infections can cause mastoid process tenderness and swelling (mastoiditis). The temporal bone consists of several parts and features:

- The **external acoustic meatus** opens into the petrous tympanic bone. It leads to, and permits examination of, the tympanic membrane (**Figure 8.8**)
- The **squamous part** (flattened) forms the lower lateral part of the cranial vault around the ear region
- The **mastoid process** is the rounded bony mass located posterior to the ear lobule, where its apex is palpable. It contains air cells that communicate with the middle ear

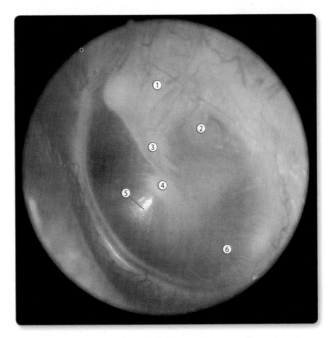

Figure 8.8 Otoscopic view of the left tympanic membrane. ① Flaccid part of tympanic membrane, ② projection of long process of incus, ③ handle of malleus, ④ umbo, ⑤ cone of light (points antero-inferiorly), ⑥ tense part of tympanic membrane.

- The **zygomatic process** projects anteriorly from just in front of the upper tragus. It joins the temporal process of the zygoma to form the zygomatic arch, which marks the level of the middle cranial fossa floor

Suprameatal triangle

The suprameatal triangle is a useful surgical marker for the surface position of the mastoid/tympanic antrum of the middle ear (**Figures 8.6** and **8.7**). The triangle is bordered:

- **Superiorly** by a line parallel to the superior border of the zygomatic arch
- **Posteriorly** by a vertical line through the posterior border of the external acoustic meatus
- **Anteroinferiorly** by the posterosuperior margin of the external acoustic meatus

Occipital bone

The occipital bone forms the posterior and inferior part of the cranial vault (**Figures 8.6** and **8.7**). The external occipital protuberance (inion) is a palpable midline projection that marks the point at which the sagittal, straight and transverse dural venous sinuses converge within the cranium (**Figures 8.9** and **8.11**). The superior nuchal lines are palpable ridges of bone, which pass laterally from the protuberance and serve as muscle and ligament attachment points.

Infant skull and fontanelles

The infant skull has a relatively small viscerocranium compared to the neurocranium. The infant calvaria is

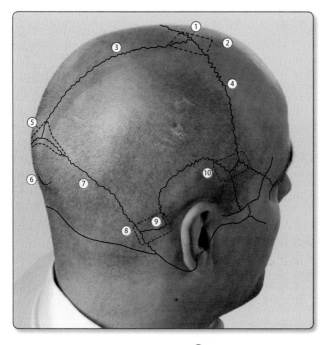

Figure 8.9 Sutures and fontanelles of the skull. (1) Site of anterior fontanelle (infant)/bregma (adult), (2) superior sagittal sinus, (3) sagittal suture, (4) coronal suture, (5) site of posterior fontanelle (infant)/lambda (adult), (6) inion (external occipital protuberance), (7) lambdoid suture, (8) site of posterolateral mastoid fontanelle (infant)/asterion (adult), (9) parietomastoid suture, (10) site of anterolateral sphenoidal fontanelle (infant)/pterion (adult).

relatively soft and mobile due to the presence of membranous joints, which enable skull remodelling during neural growth. Several large joints known as fontanelles form soft spots on the infant skull (**Table 8.1**), which are represented as palpable features on the adult skull (**Figure 8.9**).

Fontanelle	Location	Adult formation and location
Anterior	Anteriorly between frontal and parietal bones	Bregma (anterior calvarium at highest point of coronal suture)
Posterior	Posteriorly between parietal and occipital bones	Lambda (7–10 cm superior to the inion)
Mastoid	Lower temporal region posterior to ear	Asterion (posterosuperior to the mastoid)
Sphenoid	Anterior temporal region	Pterion (4 cm superior to midpoint of zygomatic arch)

Table 8.1 Fontanelles of the infant cranium and their adult formations.

8.2 Intracranial structures

Reference lines of the cranium

Standardised marker lines can be used to approximate the position of key intracranial structures (**Table 8.2** and **Figure 8.10**)

Line	Course	Features marked
Nasion–inion	Across the calvaria, from the nasion anteriorly to the inion posteriorly	Superior sagittal sinus; falx cerebri; longitudinal fissure of the brain
Reid baseline (Frankfurt plane)	Through inferior margin of the orbit and upper margin of the external acoustic meatus	Standard horizontal radiographic baseline of the skull; floor of middle cranial fossa
Condylar	Vertically through the mandibular condyle, perpendicular to Reid's baseline	Plane of anteriormost extent of central sulcus of brain
Mastoid (posterior auricular)	Vertically through the midpoint of the mastoid process perpendicular to Reid's baseline	Plane of posteriormost extent of lateral (Sylvian) sulcus of brain

Table 8.2 Reference lines of the cranium and underlying features.

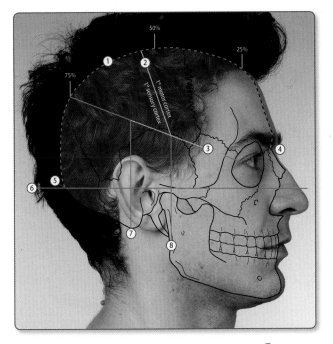

Figure 8.10 Reference lines of the cranium and sulci of the brain. (1) Nasion-inion line divided into quarters, (2) central sulcus of the brain, (3) line from lateral canthus of eye to 75% point on nasion–inion line, green section marks lateral (Sylvian) sulcus of brain, (4) nasion, (5) inion, (6) Reid's (Frankfurt) baseline, (7) mastoid/posterior auricular line, (8) condylar line.

Key brain sulci, fissures and gyri

The positions of key fissures, sulci and gyri can be mapped out using the standard reference lines of the skull (**Figure 8.11**):

- The **longitudinal fissure** runs along the nasion–inion line
- The **lateral (Sylvian) sulcus** sits along a line passing from the lateral canthus of the eye to the 75% point on the nasion–inion line and extends to the intersection with the mastoid line (**Figure 8.10**)

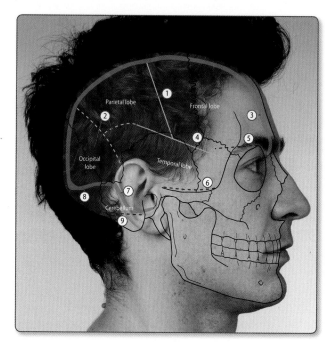

Figure 8.11 Dural venous sinuses, cranial fossae and brain lobes. ① Central sulcus, ② approximate division between lobes (hatched green lines), ③ superior sagittal sinus and position of falx cerebri, ④ lateral (Sylvian) sulcus of brain, ⑤ level of anterior cranial fossa floor (red line), ⑥ level of middle cranial fossa floor (red line), ⑦ sigmoid sinus, ⑧ transverse sinus, ⑨ level of posterior cranial fossa floor (red line).

- The **central sulcus** is approximated by drawing a line from a point ~ 2 cm posterior to the 50% point on the nasion–inion line to a point on the lateral sulcus line where it is intersected by the condylar line
- The **primary motor** and **sensory cortices** sit immediately anterior and posterior, respectively, to the central sulcus

Brain lobes, cerebellum and dural venous sinuses
The dural venous sinuses and parts of the cerebral cortex sit close to the skull therefore knowledge of their location is

essential to prevent damage, and guide positioning, during surgical access via burr hole (used to remove extradural and subdural haematomas) or craniotomy. Bony landmarks and reference lines are used to guide placement (**Table 8.3** and **Figure 8.11**)

Cranial fossae

The base/floor of the neurocranium is divided into cranial fossae, the levels of which mark the inferior extent of the brain lobes and cerebellum (**Figure 8.11**).

- The **anterior cranial fossa** sits level with the superior margin of the orbit and the pterion

Lobe/venous sinus	Surface marking
Frontal lobe	Deep to the frontal and parietal bones, anterior to the central sulcus and sat on the anterior cranial fossa floor
Temporal lobe	Deep to the temporal bone, inferior to the lateral sulcus and sat on middle cranial fossa floor
Parietal lobe	Deep to the parietal bone and posterior to the central sulcus
Occipital lobe	Deep to parietal and occipital bones and superior to the level of transverse sinus
Cerebellum	Deep to the occipital bone, inferior to the level of the transverse sinus and sat on the posterior cranial fossa floor
Superior sagittal sinus	Runs sagittally along the nasion–inion line, but can deviate to the right of the midline by up to 1 cm
Transverse sinuses	Run anteriorly from the inion to the parietomastoid suture on both the left and right sides, which is palpable posterosuperior to the mastoid
Sigmoid sinus	Curves inferiorly from the parietomastoid suture toward a point 1 cm proximal to the mastoid apex, then passes into the jugular foramen (2 cm deep to the inferior border of the external acoustic meatus)

Table 8.3 Surface markings of brain lobes and dural venous sinuses.

- The **middle cranial fossa** sits level with the upper border of the zygomatic arch
- The **posterior cranial fossa** sits level with a plane ~ 1 cm above the mastoid process apex

8.3 Muscles of the head and face

The region contains muscles for mandibular movement and facial expression (**Figure 8.12**). Despite most facial expression muscles being indistinct, knowing the location of several key muscles can help localise nerve lesions during cranial nerve examination.

Orbicularis oculi This muscle is arranged in concentric rings within both the eyelids (palpebral part) and surrounding tissues (orbital part). It is tested and palpated via eyelid closing. Paralysis leads to a dry eye or epiphora.

Orbicularis oris This muscle is arranged in concentric circles within the lips. It is used during the formation of words and to prevent the escape of food and saliva. The muscle is tested and palpated with the lips closed and pursed (kissing position). Paralysis leads to drooling/food escape from the mouth.

Modiolus This is the point of union of several facial muscles at the lateral angle of the mouth where it is felt as a firm mass (**Figure 8.12**). It can produce skin dimples when smiling. The modiolar muscles can be palpated regionally when in use and include platysma, buccinator and the muscles in **Table 8.4**.

Platysma This is a broad thin subcutaneous muscle, which passes inferolaterally across the neck from the modiolus, lower facial muscles and inferior border of the mandible (**Figure 8.13**). It blends with subcutaneous tissues of the upper thoracic and shoulder regions.

Buccinator This is a flat muscle in the cheek, which attaches to the maxillary and mandibular alveolar processes, the modiolus and pterygomandibular raphe (**Figure 8.14**). Buccinator prevents the cheeks from blowing out when whistling and helps clear the oral vestibule of food.

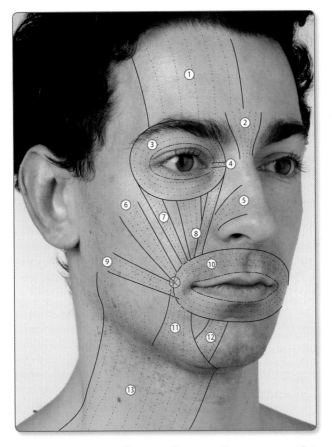

Figure 8.12 Facial muscles. ① Frontalis, ② procerus, ③ orbicularis oculi, ④ medial palpebral ligament, ⑤ nasalis, ⑥ zygomaticus major, ⑦ zygomaticus minor, ⑧ levator labii superioris, ⑨ risorius, ⑩ orbicularis oris, ⑪ depressor anguli oris, ⑫ depressor labii inferioris, ⑬ platysma, Ⓧ modiolus.

Occipitofrontalis This is formed by two muscle bellies connected by an aponeurosis that forms a layer of the scalp. Frontalis covers the anterior forehead and wrinkles the forehead, raises the eyebrows and protracts the scalp.

Muscle	Location/attachments
Zygomaticus major and minor	Pass from the lateral and anterior aspects of the zygoma to the modiolus and upper lip
Risorius	Passes posteriorly from the modiolus toward the angle of the mandible
Depressor anguli oris	Passes inferiorly from the modiolus to the mandible
Levator labii superioris	Passes from the nose and inferomedial orbital margin to the modiolus

Table 8.4 Facial muscles attached to the modiolus.

Occipitalis covers the lower part of the occipital bone above the superior nuchal line and retracts the scalp.

Masseter This muscle passes posteroinferiorly from the zygoma and anterior zygomatic arch to the lower lateral aspect of the mandibular ramus and angle. It is best seen and palpated with the teeth clenched.

Clinical insight

Blood can pass deep to the scalp aponeurosis following trauma and track to periorbital tissues producing a black/panda eye.

Temporalis This muscle passes from the temporal fossa to the mandibular coronoid process. It can be palpated via a hand placed over the lateral cranium whilst clenching the teeth.

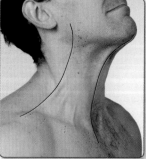

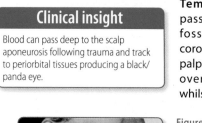

Figure 8.13 Anterolateral neck: platysma muscle.

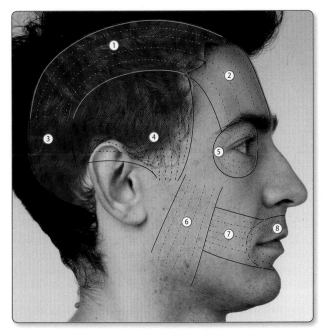

Figure 8.14 Lateral view of skull muscles. ① Epicranial aponeurosis of occipitofrontalis, ② frontalis, ③ occipitalis, ④ temporalis, ⑤ orbicularis oculi, ⑥ masseter, ⑦ buccinator, ⑧ orbicularis oris.

8.4 Nose, nasal cavity and paranasal sinuses

Nose and nasal cavity

The left and right nares open into the nasal vestibule and cavity. When looking into the nasal cavity via the nares several structures can be identified (**Figure 8.15**):

- The **nasal septa** divides the nasal cavity into left and right sides. The flexible septal cartilage protrudes anteriorly. It connects with the bony part of the nasal septum posteriorly within the nasal cavity

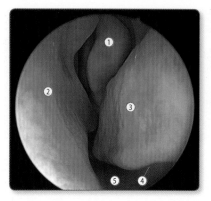

Figure 8.15 Nasal septum and conchae of the left nasal cavity. ① Middle concha, ② nasal septum, ③ inferior concha, ④ inferior meatus (covered by inferior concha), ⑤ floor of nasal cavity.

- The **nasal conchae** curl inferomedially from their attachment to the lateral nasal cavity wall. The inferior concha appears larger and closer to the nares, the middle concha appears smaller and distant and the superior concha is difficult to see
- The **meatus** are the open regions located under each concha

Clinical insight

Heavy nasal bleeds (epistaxis) often occur due to the confluence of five arterial vessels on the anteroinferior septum (Kiesselbach's plexus/Little's area).

Clinical insight

Ethmoid sinusitis can easily spread to the periorbital tissues causing optic problems via mucocele, pyocele or neuritis.

Paranasal sinuses

The frontal, maxillary, and ethmoidal sinuses are air-filled spaces located in their respective bones that mostly drain to the middle meatus of the nasal cavity (**Figures 8.16** and **8.17**). The frontal and maxillary sinuses can be inspected using transillumination via the superomedial orbital margin and hard palate/cheek, respectively. Upper respiratory tract infections can spread to the paranasal air sinuses resulting in local and referred pain via the trigeminal nerve (**Table 8.5**).

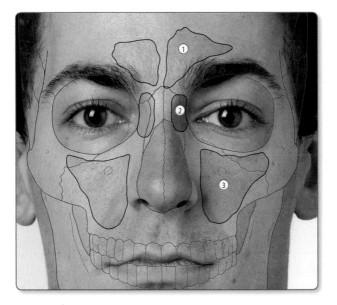

Figure 8.16 Paranasal sinuses. ① Frontal sinus, ② ethmoid sinus (air cells), ③ maxillary sinus.

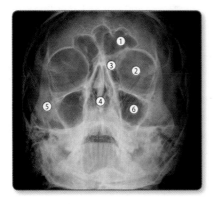

Figure 8.17 Radiograph of the face, paranasal sinuses and orbit. ① Frontal sinus, ② orbit, ③ ethmoid sinus (air cells), ④ nasal septum, ⑤ zygoma, ⑥ maxillary sinus.

Sinus	Surface location	Innervation and pain referral
Frontal	Frontal bone deep to the glabella and superciliary arches	CN Va: frontal headache; orbital/periorbital pain
Ethmoid	Between the nasal cavity and the medial orbital wall, deep to the nasal bones	
Maxillary	Body of the maxilla extending inferiorly to the alveolar process, superiorly to the orbital floor and laterally to the zygoma	CN Vb: maxillary teeth; anterior face; cheek

Table 8.5 Location and innervation of the paranasal sinuses.

8.5 Nerves

Knowledge of the position and course of the nerves of the face is important in anaesthetics, parotid/facial surgery and localising causes of nerve damage.

Cervical spinal nerves

The cervical spinal nerves have dorsal and ventral rami (branches) (**Figure 8.18**). The dorsal rami provide sensory innervation to the occipital region of the head, associated cranial dura and posterior neck. The ventral rami of C2–C4 innervate the posterolateral scalp and pinna, and the anterior and lateral neck. Compression of the C2–C3 dorsal rami can produce a posterior headache. Note, spinal nerve C1 does not innervate a dermatome.

Trigeminal nerve (CN V)

The trigeminal nerve provides sensory innervation to the skin and deep tissues of the face via three main branches (ophthalmic, maxillary and mandibular) (**Figure 8.18**). In general, the main branch innervating an area of skin also innervates structures deep to that area of skin, examples of which are shown in **Table 8.6**.

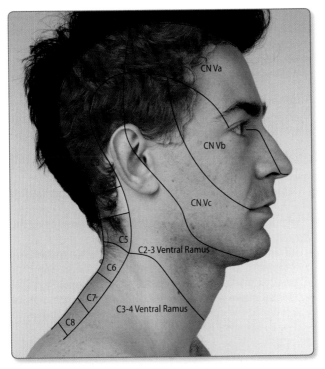

Figure 8.18 Cutaneous innervation of the head and face.

Main branch	Regions and structures innervated
Ophthalmic (CN Va)	Mucosa of the anterosuperior nasal cavity and frontal, ethmoidal and sphenoidal sinuses; frontal and ethmoid bones; conjunctiva; cornea; cranial dura
Maxillary (CN Vb)	Mucosa of the maxillary sinus, posteroinferior nasal cavity, superior oral vestibule, hard and soft palates, nasopharynx; maxillary bone, teeth and gums; cranial dura
Mandibular (CN Vc)	Mandible, teeth and gums; mucosa of the inferior oral vestibule, anterior two thirds of the tongue, floor of the mouth and oropharynx; temporomandibular joint; cranial dura; external acoustic meatus

Table 8.6 Structures innervated by the trigeminal nerve (CN V).

Pain can be referred between structures innervated by the same main branch of CN V, therefore knowledge of the structures innervated helps guide examination. For example, maxillary sinus infection may present as maxillary tooth pain, or mandibular tooth infection as temporomandibular joint pain.

Supraorbital, infraorbital and mental nerves

The terminal branches of each main branch of CN V emerge onto the face via foramina, which sit along a vertical line ~ 2.5 cm lateral to the midline (**Figures 8.19** and **8.20**). Each nerve can be blocked at their points of exit in cases of neuralgia, facial pain or herpes-zoster pain.

- **Supraorbital nerve (CN Va)** emerges from the supraorbital foramen, a palpable notch located in the superomedial margin of the orbit, and passes posterosuperiorly over the scalp towards the vertex
- **Infraorbital nerve (CN Vb)** emerges from the infraorbital foramen 1 cm below the inferior orbital margin. Branches pass to the inferior eyelid, lateral nose and upper lip
- **Mental nerve (CN Vc)** emerges from the mental foramen inferior to the apex of mandibular tooth 4 or 5 (premolar 1 or 2). Branches pass to the lower lip and chin

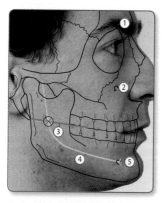

Figure 8.19 Foramen of the face and inferior alveolar nerve of the mandible. ① Supraorbital foramen, ② infraorbital foramen, ③ plane of occlusal surface of mandibular molar teeth (marks plane of mandibular foramen), ④ inferior alveolar nerve in mandibular canal, ⑤ mental nerve emerging from mental foramen, ⓧ surface position of mandibular foramen (located on deep surface of ramus).

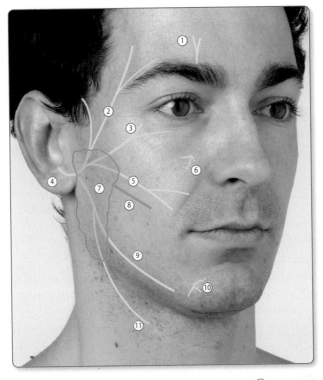

Figure 8.20 Facial and trigeminal nerves and the parotid gland. ① Supraorbital nerve (CN Va), ② facial nerve: temporal branches, ③ facial nerve: zygomatic branches, ④ facial nerve, ⑤ facial nerve: buccal branches, ⑥ infraorbital nerve (CN Vb), ⑦ parotid gland (green borders), ⑧ parotid duct, ⑨ facial nerve: marginal mandibular branches, ⑩ mental nerve (CN Vc), ⑪ facial nerve: cervical branches.

Inferior alveolar nerve

The inferior alveolar nerve (from **CN Va**) passes into the mandibular canal via the mandibular foramen on the inner surface of the ramus, approximately halfway between the inferior border and the notch (**Figure 8.19**). When anaesthetising the nerve via the oral cavity the level of the foramen is approximated by a plane running parallel to, or just above, the occlusal surfaces of the mandibular molar teeth.

Facial nerve (CN VII)

The facial nerve emerges deep to the mastoid process and passes anteroinferiorly through the midpoint of a triangle drawn between the mastoid, the mandibular angle and the temporomandibular joint to enter the parotid gland within which it divides into five branches that innervate the muscles of facial expression (**Figure 8.20** and **Table 8.7**).

Clinical insight

Newborn infants have an underdeveloped mastoid process, putting them at risk of facial nerve compression (where it exits the skull) during forceps delivery.

8.6 Viscera

Submandibular gland

The submandibular salivary gland sits in the posterior part of the submandibular triangle and is palpable as a firm mass on

Branch	Exit point from parotid	Route/surface marking
Temporal	Superior border	Along a line passing from the ear lobule to a point ~ 2 cm superior to the lateral eyebrow
Zygomatic	Superior/upper anterior border	Anteriorly above the parotid duct toward the inferior eyelid and lateral nose
Buccal	Anterior border (upper-middle part)	Anteriorly along a similar line as the parotid duct, either above or below it
Marginal mandibular	Lower anterior/ inferior border	Along the inferior mandibular border, or ~ 1–2 cm inferior to it, towards the chin
Cervical	Inferior border	Emerges ~ 1 cm inferior to mandibular angle; travels anteroinferiorly into the neck

Table 8.7 Surface marking/routes of the five branches of the facial nerve.

the inner surface of the mandibular body, near to its angle (**Figure 8.21**). Note, the gland is easily confused for an enlarged submandibular lymph node.

Parotid gland

The parotid gland (serous salivary) is situated on the lateral face (**Figure 8.21**). Its borders can be mapped out as follows:

- The **superior border** sits inferior to the zygomatic arch. It passes anteriorly from the temporomandibular joint to the posterior border of masseter, level with, or ~ 1–2 cm below, the zygomatic arch

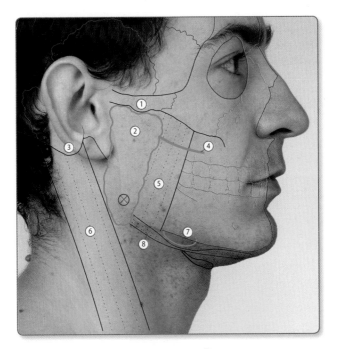

Figure 8.21 Parotid and submandibular glands. ① Zygomatic arch, ② parotid gland, ③ mastoid process, ④ parotid duct, ⑤ masseter, ⑥ sternocleidomastoid, ⑦ submandibular gland, ⑧ digastric (posterior belly), Ⓧ position of mandibular angle.

- The **anterior border** follows and overlaps the posterior border of masseter and then passes over the mandibular angle to meet the anterior border of sternocleidomastoid
- The **posterior border** ascends sternocleidomastoid to the mastoid process and then clasps the posterior and medial surfaces of the mandibular ramus as it ascends toward the temporomandibular joint. Large parotid tumours can therefore protrude into the oropharynx or oral cavity

> **Clinical insight**
>
> Parotid stones present as a hard lumps in the gland or along the course of the duct.

Parotid duct

The parotid duct drains the gland into the oral vestibule. The duct exits the gland's anterior border and travels along a line passing from the tragus of the ear to the lateral angle of the mouth or just superior to it (**Figure 8.21**). It opens into the oral vestibule opposite the upper 2nd molar tooth (**Figure 8.22**). The duct opening can be inspected for purulent discharge in suspected parotitis and can be cannulated to enable radiographic investigation (sialography).

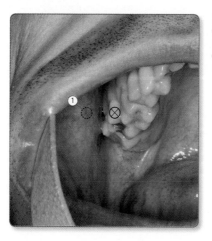

Figure 8.22 Parotid duct. ① Opening of parotid duct into oral vestibule, ⓧ 2nd maxillary (upper) molar tooth.

Eye region

Eyelid

The eyelids are formed by connective tissue plates (tarsi) covered externally by skin and internally by conjunctiva (**Figure 8.23**). The medial and lateral palpebral ligaments attach the tarsi to the orbital margins. Tightly closing the eye allows the medial ligament to be felt as a firm horizontal band passing to a bony tubercle. The ligament marks the position of the underlying lacrimal sac.

Cornea and sclera

The cornea is the clear convex avascular covering of the anterior eye (**Figure 8.23**). The iris, pupil and fundus can be examined

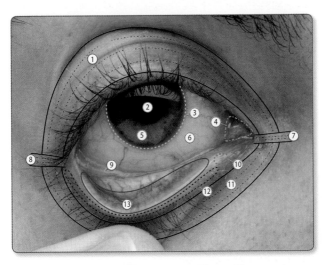

Figure 8.23 Eye and eyelids. ① Superior tarsus, ② pupil, ③ margin of cornea, ④ region of lacrimal lake covering lacrimal caruncle, ⑤ iris, ⑥ sclera, ⑦ medial palpebral ligament, ⑧ lateral palpebral ligament, ⑨ inferior conjunctival fornix, ⑩ lacrimal punctum on the lacrimal papilla, ⑪ inferior tarsus, ⑫ region of openings of the ciliary glands and of sty formation (black dotted line), ⑬ Location of tarsal glands and of tarsal chalazion formation (red line).

via the cornea. The sclera is the white part of the eyeball that is covered in conjunctiva. Conjunctival blood vessels can become prominent and dilated when inflamed.

Lacrimal, tarsal and ciliary glands

Several glands secrete into the region (**Figures 8.23** and **8.24**):

- The **lacrimal gland** (tear fluid) has orbital and palpebral parts and is located in the superolateral orbit under the eyelid
- The **tarsal glands** (lipid) are located on the inner surfaces of the upper and lower eyelids and are seen as parallel rows

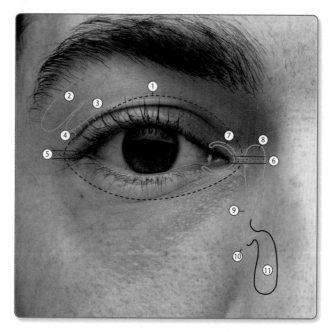

Figure 8.24 Lacrimal gland and lacrimal duct system. (1) Projection of position of conjunctival fornix, (2) lacrimal gland: orbital part, (3) lacrimal gland: palpebral part, (4) lacrimal gland ducts, (5) Lateral palpebral ligament, (6) medial palpebral ligament overlying lacrimal sac, (7) lacrimal canaliculi, (8) lacrimal sac, (9) nasolacrimal duct, (10) nasolacrimal duct opening in the inferior meatus of nasal cavity, (11) inferior concha of nasal cavity.

of yellow rectangles. Infection produces a mass behind the eyelid, a tarsal chalazion, that rubs on the eyeball
- The **ciliary glands** (sebaceous) sit at the base of the eyelid hairs. Infection produces a red swelling known as a sty

Conjunctival sac and fornix

The conjunctival sac is located between the conjunctiva of the eyelid and of the outer facing surface of the eye (**Figure 8.23**). The conjunctival fornix represents the point at which the conjunctiva reflect from the eye to the eyelid. The fornix sits up to 1 cm from the edge of the eyelid and is a region where foreign debris and contact lenses can become trapped. The fornix can be viewed by retracting the eyelid.

Lacrimal duct system

Tear fluid is drained from the lacrimal lake to the nasal cavity via a duct system (**Figure 8.24**), which can get blocked by infection, trauma

> **Clinical insight**
>
> Direct eyeball trauma can produce hyphema, a visible collection of blood between the cornea and iris.

or nasal cavity tumour/polyps resulting in epiphora.
- The **lacrimal punctum** is a small hole located on the raised lacrimal papilla of the medial part of each eyelid. They open into the lacrimal canaliculi, which pass medially to the lacrimal sac
- The **lacrimal sac** sits deep to the medial palpebral ligament, where it can be massaged inferiorly in cases of blockage
- The **nasolacrimal duct** passes inferolaterally from the lacrimal sac along a line from the medial palpebral ligament toward the premolar teeth and drains into the inferior meatus of the nasal cavity, ~ 2–3 cm posterior to the nares. In children a nasolacrimal duct cyst (dacryocystocele) is seen as a blue swelling of the skin covering the duct

8.7 Oral cavity and oral vestibule

The mouth is bordered by the hard palate, alveolar processes, teeth and palatal/faucial arches. The oral cavity is the main area housing the tongue and the oral vestibule is the narrow area located between the cheeks, lips, teeth and alveolar processes.

Teeth

The maxillary and mandibular teeth are located in the alveolar processes of the maxilla and mandible (**Figure 8.25**). Adults

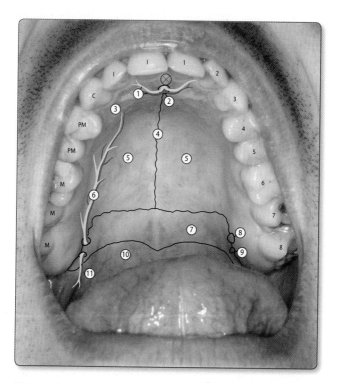

Figure 8.25 Teeth and the hard and soft palates. ① Nasopalatine nerve and greater palatine artery, ② incisive fossa/canal, ③ maxillary alveolar process, ④ palatine raphe overlying intermaxillary suture, ⑤ palatine process of maxilla (hard palate), ⑥ greater palatine artery and nerve, ⑦ horizontal plate of palatine bone (hard palate), ⑧ greater palatine foramen, ⑨ lesser palatine foramen, ⑩ soft palate, ⑪ lesser palatine artery and nerve, ⓧ incisive papilla, teeth are numbered 1-8 from anterior to posterior or named, I, incisor, C, canine, PM, premolar, M, molar.

have up to 32 teeth, eight per side and level of the mouth, which are numbered 1–8 from anterior to posterior. The normal adult arrangement from anterior to posterior being 2 incisors, 1 canine, 2 premolars and 3 molars.

Palate
Hard palate

The hard palate is formed anteriorly by the palatine processes of the left and right maxilla and posteriorly by the palatine bone (horizontal part) (**Figure 8.25**). The whole palate is covered in firm ridged mucosa. The maxillary palatine processes join at a midline raphe. Failure to join during development results in visible midline clefting, which can be accompanied by clefting of the top lip.

Palatine foramen and neurovasculature

The foramen of the palate transmit sensory nerves that innervate the palate, associated alveolar processes and teeth (**Figure 8.25**). They can be anaesthetised at their point of entry onto the palate during oral/dental procedures.

- The **greater** and **lesser palatine foramen** are located ~ 1 cm medial to the 3rd maxillary molar tooth, in the palatine bone. The greater is anterior to the lesser. They transmit the greater and lesser palatine nerves and vessels
- The **incisive fossa** and **canal** are located in the midline immediately posterior to the central incisor teeth and the incisive papilla, a raised midline piece of mucosa. The fossa marks the end of the incisive canal, which transmits the nasopalatine nerve and greater palatine artery

Soft palate

The fibromuscular soft palate attaches to the posterior of the hard palate and hangs posteroinferiorly into the oropharynx (**Figure 8.26**). The uvula projects inferiorly in the midline. Movement of the soft palate is assessed during cranial nerve testing. The soft palate deviates away from the side of a vagus nerve (CN X) lesion.

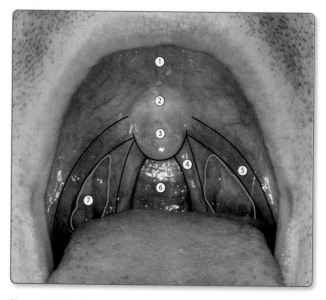

Figure 8.26 Palatal arches, oropharynx, uvula and palatine tonsils. ① Palatine raphe (hard palate), ② soft palate, ③ uvula, ④ palatopharyngeal arch, ⑤ palatoglossal arch, ⑥ posterior wall of oropharynx, ⑦ location of palatine tonsil (green border).

Palatoglossal and palatopharyngeal arches

The palatoglossal and palatopharyngeal (faucial) arches are located between the oral cavity and oropharynx and are formed by muscles sitting under the mucosa (**Figure 8.26**). The palatoglossal arch sits anterolateral to the palatopharyngeal arch. The indented region between the arches, the tonsillar fossa, houses the lymphoid palatine tonsils, which are covered in visible mucosal crypts (indentations). The tonsils can become infected or develop tonsiloliths, which cause halitosis.

Floor of the mouth
Sublingual fold

The mucosa under the tongue is folded to form the midline lingual frenulum (**Figure 8.27**). Two additional mucosal folds,

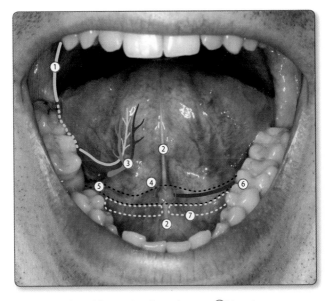

Figure 8.27 Floor of the mouth and ventral tongue. (1) Lingual nerve, (2) lingual frenulum, (3) deep lingual artery and vein, (4) sublingual caruncle with opening of submandibular duct (orange border), (5) sublingual folds (black border), (6) sublingual duct, (7) sublingual glands (pink border).

the left and right sublingual folds, run posterolaterally from the lingual frenulum. Each fold:

- Marks the line of travel of the submandibular duct
- Contains the sublingual glands, the ducts of which open on to the fold
- Posterolaterally marks the position of the lingual nerve passing close to the root of tooth 8

The submandibular ducts open on to the raised sublingual caruncle at the point where the sublingual fold intersects the frenulum. The duct is a common place for stone formation (sialolithiasis), which may be palpable within the duct, painful or painless. Infection of the sublingual gland can cause regional pain and swelling.

Lingual nerve

The sensory lingual nerve (from CN Vc) travels into the floor of the mouth close to the root of the 3rd mandibular molar tooth, where it is palpable and vulnerable to damage during tooth extraction. The posterolateral extent of the sublingual fold is a useful marker of the nerves position. It then continues toward the tip of the tongue alongside the deep lingual artery and vein, which are visible on the ventral tongue.

8.8 Neck

Triangles of the neck

For descriptive purposes the neck can be divided into triangles, the borders of which are formed by muscles and bone. The two main triangles of the neck are the anterior and the posterior.

Anterior triangle and its subdivisions

The anterior triangle (**Figure 8.28**), or anterior cervical region, is bordered:

- Posteriorly by sternocleidomastoid
- Superiorly by the inferior border of the mandible
- Anteriorly by the midline

The anterior triangle can be further subdivided into four triangles (**Table 8.8**).

Muscles of the anterior triangle

- **Sternocleidomastoid** is a prominent muscle that passes from the mastoid process and superior nuchal line to the manubrium (sternal head) and the medial third of the clavicle (clavicular head). It is best seen and palpated with the head in resisted axial rotation
- **Digastric** has two bellies united by a tendon. It can be mapped between three points, the inferior border of the midline chin, the lateral part of the hyoid body and the mastoid process. The superior belly runs between the first two points and the inferior belly between the latter two

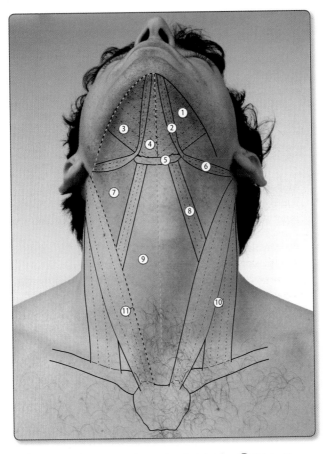

Figure 8.28 Anterior triangle of the neck and subdivisions. ① Mylohyoid, ② anterior belly of digastric, ③ submandibular triangle (green), ④ submental triangle (orange), ⑤ body of hyoid bone, ⑥ posterior belly of digastric, ⑦ carotid triangle (red), ⑧ superior belly of omohyoid, ⑨ muscular triangle (blue), ⑩ sternocleidomastoid (sternal and clavicular heads), ⑪ border of the right anterior triangle of neck (blue dashed line).

Triangle	Borders
Submandibular	Anterior and posterior bellies of digastric; inferior border of the mandible
Submental	Anterior bellies of digastric (left and right); body of the hyoid
Carotid	Posterior belly of digastric; sternocleidomastoid; superior belly of omohyoid
Muscular	Superior belly of omohyoid; sternocleidomastoid; midline

Table 8.8 Subdivisions of the anterior triangle of the neck.

- **Mylohyoid** forms the floor of the mouth and sits within the submental and submandibular triangles. It passes from the inner surface of the mandible to a midline raphe and the hyoid bone
- **Omohyoid** has two bellies united by a tendon. The superior belly passes along a line that runs from the lateral part of the hyoid body to a point approximately one third of the way up sternocleidomastoid, from its sternal attachment. The inferior belly passes through the posterior triangle

Posterior triangle and subdivisions

The posterior triangle of the neck (**Figure 8.29**), or lateral cervical region, is bordered:
- **Medially** by sternocleidomastoid
- **Posteriorly** by trapezius
- **Inferiorly** by the clavicle

The posterior triangle can be subdivided into two parts by the inferior belly of the omohyoid muscle (**Table 8.9**).

Muscles of the posterior triangle

- **Inferior belly of omohyoid** crosses the lower part of the posterior triangle along a line passing from the cricoid cartilage to the medial edge of the trapezius attachment to the clavicle
- **Scalene muscles** (**anterior, medius** and **posterior**) (**Figure 8.30**) are located in the floor of the posterior triangle and can be felt as a hard mass passing inferolaterally from the lateral border of sternocleidomastoid. The almost vertical groove between scalenus anterior and medius is a useful marker for

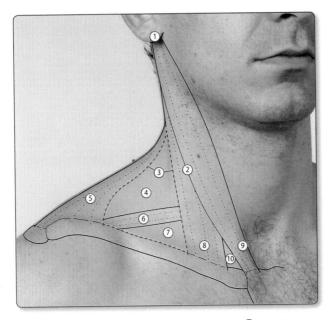

Figure 8.29 Posterior triangle of the neck and subdivisions. ① Mastoid process, ② sternocleidomastoid, ③ borders of right posterior triangle of neck (blue dashed line), ④ occipital triangle (blue), ⑤ trapezius, ⑥ inferior belly of omohyoid, ⑦ omoclavicular/supraclavicular triangle (green), ⑧ clavicular head of sternocleidomastoid, ⑨ sternal head of sternocleidomastoid, ⑩ lesser supraclavicular fossa (overlying internal jugular vein).

Triangle	Borders
Occipital	Trapezius; sternocleidomastoid; inferior belly of omohyoid
Supraclavicular/omoclavicular	Inferior belly of omohyoid; clavicle; sternocleidomastoid

Table 8.9 Subdivisions of the posterior triangle of the neck.

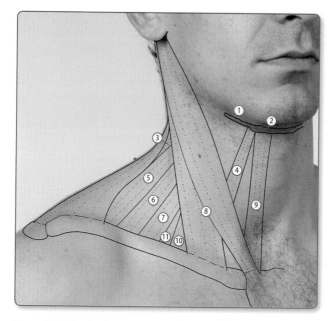

Figure 8.30 Muscles of posterior triangle of the neck. ① Greater horn of hyoid, ② body of hyoid, ③ splenius capitis, ④ superior belly of omohyoid (inferior belly not shown), ⑤ levator scapulae, ⑥ scalenus posterior, ⑦ scalenus medius, ⑧ sternocleidomastoid, ⑨ sternohyoid, ⑩ scalenus anterior, ⑪ interscalene groove (point of emergence of brachial plexus and subclavian artery).

brachial plexus localisation and interscalene plexus block. It can be palpated level with the cricoid cartilage on the lateral border of sternocleidomastoid

Greater and lesser supraclavicular fossae The lesser supraclavicular fossa is the small triangular indented region located between the clavicular and sternal heads of sternocleidomastoid. Its superior apex marks an access point for internal jugular vein cannulation. The greater supraclavicular fossa is the indentation located above the clavicle over the region of the supraclavicular triangle. The subclavian vessels and brachial plexus pass through the region and can be palpated there.

8.9 Neurovasculature

Nerves

Multiple nerves pass across the neck in both superficial and deep positions (**Figure 8.31** and **8.32**). Nerves must be identified and preserved, especially during surgical neck dissection and lymph node clearance. The cervical and brachial plexi can be anaesthetised in the neck to enable neck or upper limb procedures, respectively.

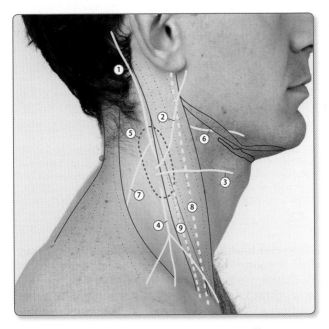

Figure 8.31 Nerves and nerve point of the neck (lateral view). ① Lesser occipital nerve, ② greater auricular nerve, ③ transverse cervical nerve, ④ supraclavicular nerve, ⑤ nerve point of neck (purple hatched line), ⑥ hypoglossal nerve in carotid triangle, ⑦ accessory nerve, ⑧ course of vagus nerve in carotid sheath, ⑨ course of phrenic nerve passing between sternocleidomastoid and scalenus anterior.

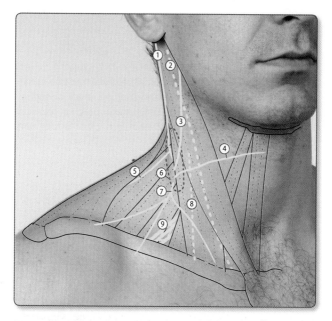

Figure 8.32 Nerves and nerve point of the neck (anterior view). ① Lesser occipital nerve, ② course of vagus nerve in carotid sheath, ③ greater auricular nerve, ④ transverse cervical nerve, ⑤ accessory nerve, ⑥ nerve point of neck (purple), ⑦ supraclavicular nerve, ⑧ course of phrenic nerve passing between sternocleidomastoid and scalenus anterior, ⑨ brachial plexus (upper trunk).

Cutaneous branches of the cervical plexus These emerge from the posterior border of the middle third of sternocleidomastoid (the nerve point of the neck), where they can be anaesthetised. They innervate skin of the scalp, neck and upper thorax. The branches and their routes of travel are shown in **Table 8.10**.

Spinal accessory nerve This emerges from a point one third to one half of the way down the posterior border of sternocleidomastoid and passes across the posterior triangle to a point approximately two thirds of the way down trapezius.

Nerve(s)	Route/surface marking
Lesser occipital	Posterosuperiorly along the posterior border of sternocleidomastoid toward the occipital region
Greater auricular	Superiorly over sternocleidomastoid toward the angle of the mandible ~ 1 cm posterior to the external jugular vein
Transverse cervical	Horizontally over sternocleidomastoid toward the laryngeal prominence; some branches travel toward the mandible
Supraclavicular	Inferolaterally and branches; some branches pass over trapezius and some over the clavicle onto the anterior thorax

Table 8.10 Surface marking/route of the cutaneous branches of the cervical plexus.

Brachial plexus (superior trunk C5 and C6) This passes inferolaterally through the posterior triangle along a line joining the laryngeal prominence to the midpoint of the clavicle. The plexus sits posterior and superior to the subclavian artery, which is palpable just medial to the midclavicular point. The plexus can be anesthetised in the posterior triangle as it passes between scalenus anterior and posterior, or around the midclavicular point

Phrenic nerve This emerges from between scalenus anterior and medius, level with the laryngeal prominence and travels inferiorly across the anterior border of scalenus anterior. It can be inadvertently anaesthetised during brachial plexus block causing diaphragmatic hemiparalysis and shortness of breath.

Vagus nerve (CN X) This nerve runs down the neck in the carotid sheath posterior, or lateral, to the carotid artery.

Hypoglossal nerve This passes through the carotid triangle, inferior to the posterior belly of digastric muscle, then passes anterosuperiorly into the submandibular triangle above mylohyoid. It is at risk during carotid endarterectomy or submandibular gland procedures.

Arteries

Many arteries pass through the head and neck (**Figure 8.33**). Knowledge of their position enables examination of pulsation, surgical access (carotid endarterectomy) and avoidance during local procedures (nerve block).

Subclavian artery

The subclavian artery passes posterior to the clavicular head of sternocleidomastoid. It often ascends above the upper level of the medial clavicle before passing inferolaterally to the upper limb. Pulsations can be palpated via the supraclavicular triangle, just medial to the midclavicular point and the cord-like structure of the brachial plexus can be palpated posteriorly. The vertebral artery, internal thoracic artery and thyrocervical trunk branch from the subclavian posterior to the sternal end of the clavicle.

Suprascapular and transverse cervical arteries

Both vessels arise ~ 2–3 cm above the sternal end of the clavicle and pass over the brachial plexus and across the posterior triangle. They are at risk of damage during brachial plexus block.

- The **transverse cervical artery** passes toward a point two thirds of the way down trapezius
- The **suprascapular artery** passes posterolaterally along the line of the clavicle toward the point of intersection between the superior scapula border and a plane passing along the medial border of the coracoid process

Common carotid arteries and carotid bifurcation

Common carotid artery This artery travels superiorly through the neck, lateral to the trachea and larynx where its pulsation can be felt against the transverse processes of C4–C6. It travels along a line passing from the sternoclavicular joint to the mandibular angle, and sits deep to sternocleidomastoid inferiorly and medial to both it and the internal jugular vein superiorly. The latter relationship provides a route of approach for carotid endarterectomy.

Carotid bifurcation The common carotid artery bifurcates at vertebral level C3–C4 (hyoid body/thyrohyoid membrane). The

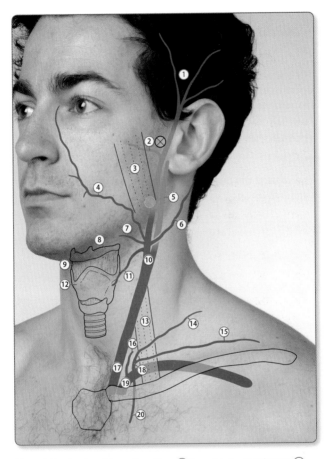

Figure 8.33 Arteries of the neck and face. ① Superficial temporal artery, ②
maxillary artery (deep to mandibular notch/upper ramus), ③ masseter, ④ facial
artery, ⑤ internal carotid artery, ⑥ occipital artery, ⑦ lingual artery, ⑧ greater
horn of the hyoid, ⑨ thyrohyoid membrane (vertebral level C4), ⑩ carotid
bifurcation, ⑪ superior thyroid artery, ⑫ laryngeal prominence (vertebral
level C5), ⑬ scalenus anterior, ⑭ transverse cervical artery, ⑮ suprascapular
artery, ⑯ vertebral artery, ⑰ common carotid artery, ⑱ thyrocervical trunk,
⑲ subclavian artery, ⑳ internal thoracic artery, Ⓧ position of mandibular
notch, Ⓧ position of mandibular angle.

carotid sinus, located just superior to the bifurcation, can be massaged to slow heart rate or to test unexplained syncope.

External carotid artery

The external carotid passes superiorly from the carotid bifurcation at C3–C4 deep to the posterior border of the mandibular ramus. It gives rise to multiple branches, which have a positional relationship to the greater horn of the hyoid (**Table 8.11** and **Figure 8.33**).

Veins

The veins of the neck can be inspected during cardiovascular examination and can be cannulated (**Figure 8.34**).

Artery	Level of origin	Route/surface marking
Superior thyroid	Below the hyoid	Passes anteroinferiorly toward the superior pole of the thyroid gland; related to external laryngeal nerve; requires ligation in thyroidectomy
Lingual	Level with the hyoid	Passes anteriorly into the floor of the mouth
Facial	Just above hyoid level	Passes onto the face just anterior to masseter where its pulsations are felt, then passes toward the angle of the mouth and then the medial eye
Occipital		Passes posterior to the mastoid process into the occipital region; pulsations are palpable 3–5 cm lateral to the inion
Maxillary	Deep to the mandibular neck	Passes anteriorly through the infratemporal fossa, deep to the mandibular notch/ramus; at risk during CN Vb/Vc nerve block
Superficial temporal		Passes superiorly onto the temporal region; pulsations are felt just anterior to the upper pinna; affected by temporal arteritis, which is diagnosed via biopsy

Table 8.11 Surface marking/route of the branches of the external carotid artery.

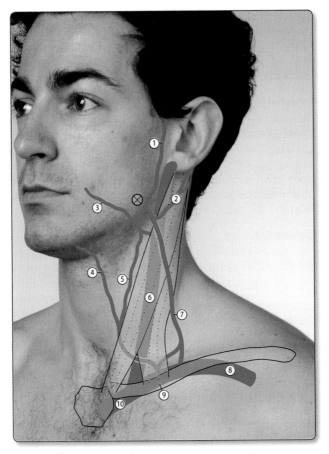

Figure 8.34 Superficial and deep veins of the neck and face. ① Retromandibular vein, ② posterior auricular vein, ③ facial vein, ④ anterior jugular vein, ⑤ communicating vein, ⑥ internal jugular vein, ⑦ external jugular vein, ⑧ axillary vein, ⑨ subclavian vein, ⑩ left brachiocephalic vein, Ⓧ position of mandibular angle.

External jugular vein

This vein passes along a line from the angle of the mandible to a point just lateral to where sternocleidomastoid joins the clavicle. It can be visualised when performing the Valsalva manoeuvre. With the patient at a 15–30° incline, the height of the blood column in the jugular veins (internal or external) relates to right atrial pressure, with rises in height indicating pathology.

Internal jugular vein

This vein passes inferiorly through the neck deep to sterno-cleidomastoid and along a line joining a point just medial to the mandibular angle/ramus to the sternal end of the clavicle. Jugular venous pulse can be examined in the vessel and recognised by its double undulation. The vein can be cannulated via the apex of the lesser supraclavicular fossa or at a point just lateral to the carotid pulse.

Subclavian vein

This vein arches through the supraclavicular triangle, posterior the clavicular head of sternocleidomastoid. It joins the internal jugular vein posterior to the sternal end of the clavicle/sternoclavicular joint to form the brachiocephalic vein. It is accessed via a point inferior to the junction between the middle third and medial third of the clavicle, and the needle aimed toward the sternal notch.

> ### Clinical insight
>
> Venous air embolus can accompany external jugular vein laceration since air is drawn into the vein during the decrease in intrathoracic pressure whilst inhaling.

8.10 Viscera

Larynx and trachea

The larynx and trachea are located superficially in the anterior midline of neck (**Figure 8.35**). Knowledge of their key features enables safe airway establishment via cricothyrotomy, tracheotomy or endotracheal intubation. The main features include:

- The **body of the hyoid** marks vertebral level C3 and can be located by running a finger posteriorly along the submental triangle until a firm midline mass is felt. The greater horns of the hyoid can be felt posterosuperiorly from the body

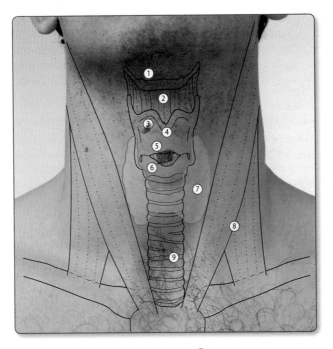

Figure 8.35 Larynx, trachea and thyroid gland. ① Body of hyoid, ② thyrohyoid membrane, ③ thyroid cartilage lamina, ④ laryngeal prominence, ⑤ cricothyroid membrane, ⑥ cricoid cartilage, ⑦ thyroid gland with isthmus crossing midline, ⑧ sternocleidomastoid, ⑨ trachea.

- The **thyrohyoid membrane** passes between the hyoid and thyroid cartilages. It sits in the palpable depression above the laryngeal prominence and marks the level of vertebra C4 and of the carotid bifurcation/sinus
- The **paired thyroid cartilage laminae** join in the anterior midline to form the raised laryngeal prominence, which marks vertebral level C5 and houses the vocal folds
- The **cricothyroid membrane** sits between the thyroid and cricoid cartilages. It is felt as a soft depression and serves as the access point for cricothyrotomy

- The **cricoid cartilage** forms a firm smooth ring below the cricothyroid membrane. It marks vertebral level C6
- The **trachea** passes inferiorly down the midline from the cricoid, where it is easily palpable. A tracheostomy accesses the trachea at the sternal notch, retraction of the thyroid isthmus is often required

Laryngeal inlet

The laryngeal inlet can be viewed with a laryngeal mirror (**Figure 8.36**). Knowledge of its normal arrangement and features enables competent examination and safe introduction of an endotracheal tube.

Thyroid gland

The thyroid gland has two lobes located on the anterolateral sides of the larynx and trachea between vertebral levels C5–T1 (thyroid cartilage just above sternal notch) (**Figure 8.35**). The isthmus joins the lobes over the 2nd and 3rd tracheal cartilages. During development the thyroid descends through the midline anterior neck via the thyroglossal duct. Cysts can form on the thyroglossal duct producing midline swellings that move on swallowing and tongue protrusion.

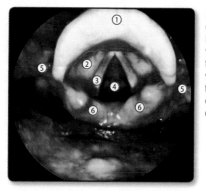

Figure 8.36 Superior view of the laryngeal inlet. (1) Epiglottis (anterior), (2) vestibular fold, (3) vocal fold, (4) rima glottidis with view of trachea, (5) piriform fossa, (6) aryepiglottic fold containing cuneiform and corniculate cartilage.

8.11 Lymphatics

Superficial nodes

Lymphatics from the head and neck drain to a series superficial nodes sat along the pericraniocervical line, external jugular vein and the region above the clavicle (**Figure 8.37**). All head and neck lymph eventually drains into deep cervical

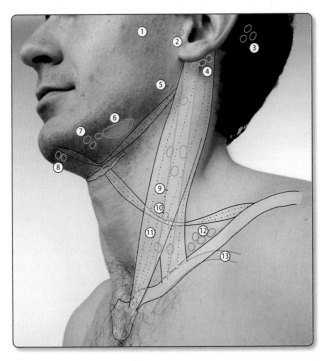

Figure 8.37 Lymph nodes of the head and neck. ① Parotid nodes, ② preauricular nodes, ③ occipital nodes, ④ mastoid nodes, ⑤ jugulodigastric node (upper deep cervical group), ⑥ submandibular gland, ⑦ submandibular nodes, ⑧ submental nodes, ⑨ internal jugular vein, ⑩ juguloomohyoid nodes (lower deep cervical group), ⑪ sternocleidomastoid, ⑫ supraclavicular nodes, ⑬ Axillary vein becoming the subclavian vein proximally.

Nodes	Location	Regions drained
Submental	Submental triangle	Chin; lip; floor of the mouth; tongue tip
Submandibular	Submandibular triangle near the facial artery	Tongue; oral cavity; lip; mandible and associated teeth; nose; lower face
Parotid/ preauricular	Lateral surface of the parotid gland anterior to the tragus	Anterior auricle; lateral scalp; forehead; upper face; eyelids; auditory meatus
Mastoid/ postauricular	Mastoid process and behind the ear	Posterolateral scalp to the vertex
Occipital	Superior nuchal line near the occipital artery	Posterior scalp; upper neck
Superficial cervical	Alongside the external jugular vein	Superficial neck tissues; mastoid and occipital nodes
Supraclavicular	Above the clavicle in the supraclavicular triangle	Superficial neck tissues; thoracic structures; foregut to left-sided nodes

Table 8.12 Location and drainage of the superficial head and cervical lymph-node groups.

nodes. Lymphadenopathy can result from head and neck infection or cancer therefore systematic examination of all node groups and knowledge of the tissues they drain is important (**Table 8.12**). The superficial nodes of the head and neck are shown in **Figure 8.37**.

Deep nodes

The deep cervical (neck) lymph nodes sit along the internal jugular vein, mostly deep to sternocleidomastoid. They are often separated into upper and lower groups (by omohyoid) or superior, middle and inferior groups according to their relative positions. Two groups of deep cervical nodes can also be defined by their relationship to the digastric and omohyoid muscles (**Table 8.13**).

Nodes	Location	Regions drained
Jugulodigastric (upper group)	Where digastric crosses the internal jugular vein	Palatine tonsil; pharynx; larynx; oral cavity; superficial node groups
Jugulo-omohyoid (lower group)	Where omohyoid crosses the internal jugular vein	Tongue; superficial node groups; upper deep cervical nodes

Table 8.13 Location and drainage of the deep cervical lymph node groups.

The jugulodigastric nodes are often felt as a firm mass posterior to the mandibular angle, and can be unequal in size when comparing left side to right, especially following upper respiratory tract infection.

Index

Note: Page numbers in **bold** or *italic* refer to tables or figures respectively.